Working in the Community 2: Practice Studies

All human knowledge takes the form of interpretation

Walter Benjamin

Working in the Community 2:

Practice Studies

First edition 2010

ISBN 978-1-4461-3908-0

Published in the USA by Lulu Press, Morrsiville, North Carolina, 27560

Table of Content

The challenge of modernity is to live without illusions
and without becoming disillusioned.

Antonio Gramsci

About This Book

> Education either functions as an instrument which is used to facilitate the integration of generations into the logic of the present system and bring about conformity to it, or it becomes 'the practice of freedom', the means by which men and women deal critically and creatively with reality and discover how to participate in the transformation of their world.
>
> Paulo Freire

This book is a companion to Working in the Community: perspective for change (Purcell 2005), which was written as a discussion of ideas that underpin professional work in community settings. The target audience for both books include both paid and unpaid workers, community activists, students and professionals operating across the range of welfare, health and education sectors.

Exploring ideas and theories about practice is of course essential to developing a critical praxis. However, ideas and theories are difficult to apply in practice. Often we find that ideas sit in splendid isolation to what actually takes place out in the community under the name of professional practice. The purpose of this second book in the Working in the Community series is to explore what actually happens in practice, what is good about it and what is not so good. The ideas from the first book, plus new conceptualisations of practice, inform these discussions.

The aim of this book is therefore to give a flavour of the range of practice out there. The examples in the book are drawn from Scotland but are equally valid, despite some policy and organisational differences for the rest of the UK and Ireland. These studies will also have relevance for practitioners in other countries. The studies are not presented as idealised examples of good practice. Each study certainly contains examples of good practice and this is useful to have. The point though, is to explore the wide ranging contexts, policy orientations, dilemmas, difficulties, achievements and failures that are the everyday experience of practitioners. These studies are practice as it is, warts and all. I am deeply indebted to the authors of the practice studies for offering us their work in order to help other practitioners learn from their experiences.

There are 11 practice studies presented here. Each study has a brief abstract outlining the setting and purpose of the work, an extensive discussion of key aspects of the work, and a final commentary. The names of the projects, workers and individuals in the studies have been removed where required to protect confidentiality.

Briefly the practice studies cover the following activities:

Practice Study 1: Community initiative to reduce violence

Practice Study 2: Lesbian, Gay, Bisexual and Transgender Equality Network

Practice Study 3: HOPE: support to offenders, prisoners and their families

Practice Study 4: Local Authority supported youth work

Practice Study 5: Men's group: community allotment

Practice Study 6: Women's group

Practice Study 7: Sikh women and their families

Practice Study 8: Grandparents Parenting Again

Practice Study 9: Chinese community fundraising group

Practice Study 10: Community Learning and Development team focusing on community capacity building

Practice Study 11: Community Voices Training Programme

The book begins with a discussion of the nature of contemporary practice, which explores a number of critical and underlying limitations to the orientation and effectiveness of how practice is conceptualised, organised and delivered, and some suggestions of how we may choose to develop our practice. The book concludes with an overview of what the practice studies tell us and what we might do about it.

Once again my thanks to everyone who has contributed to this book. Especially the practice study authors: John Bernklow, Iain Cunningham, Carole Dick, Steven Gilfoyle, Davina Hepson, Hazel Lindsay, Sara Jane McNeil, Lisa Peet, Janice Quinn, Rosemary Robertson, Trishna Sing, Lesley Ward.

Any misunderstanding and errors are of course my sole responsibility.

Rod Purcell
University of Glasgow
May 2010

About The Contributors

> We must believe that it is the darkest before the dawn of a beautiful new world. We will see it when we believe it.
>
> Saul Alinsky

John Bernklow

John Bernklow is a retired Fire-fighter, who is currently perusing his interest in community development. He is actively involved with a local environmental group Heal the Earth in Kilmarnock, In addition John works as a men's development worker with a Rosemount Lifelong Learning a community based charitable organisation in North Glasgow. He is also studying part- time at Glasgow University undertaking an MSc in Community Development.

Iain Cunningham

Iain has been involved in community development work for more than twenty years working within a variety of organisations from Inverclyde, Lanarkshire and Renfrewshire, delivering all aspects of community learning and development programmes. These programmes included; youth work, employment and training initiatives, alternative to custody projects, community regeneration funding programmes including administration of a small grants fund. Iain's first involvement with community work came about as a volunteer while undertaking the 'Duke of Edinburgh Award Scheme' with the 'BB' and his interest grew from there. Vehicle mechanic's was his first passion before becoming fully involved with community work, where he re-trained with Glasgow University and local colleges on careers guidance and management qualifications. He currently managing a community capacity building project (Community Action Team) within Paisley Partnership Regeneration Company.

Carole Dick

Carole is a graduate from Glasgow University, with a varied background in Community Development. These experiences include children's work, youth development, working with the homeless and prostitutes, working in Africa and with Sure Start. Currently, Carole works for Sure Start as centre manager for Penicuik and the surrounding rural areas; a job with a very diverse remit. Having lived abroad most of her life since age 2, Carole has developed a passion for travelling particularly looking at different cultures, how people live and interact with one another. This has given Carole great insight, which has impacted on her own practice.

Steven Gilfoyle

Steven has a long background in training and development work through community radio. He is also well known by his stage name Steg G, and is a Scottish hip hop producer, radio DJ and record executive. He is the founder and current CEO of Powercut Productions, a hip hop label based in Glasgow, Scotland. He started his early hip hop career working with local rap acts such as BAAD Company and Sons of the Devil as their DJ and producer. His first official single was released on Devil Discs and was with a 4 piece group called Powermove (Steg G, Shoey, Freestyle Master, Jimmy P). The single (But Were Different) was the first time that that the majority of people had experienced Hip Hop music with a Scottish accent and perspective

Davina Hepson

Davina Hepson was born in Edinburgh and grew up in Paisley. When Davina left school in 1972 age fifteen she worked as a trainee Hairdresser, shop assistant and apprentice Lithographic printer. Davina made a good living working as a printer and print finisher for over twenty years. Between 1994 -1996 she studied at Glasgow's College of Building and Printing, graduating with merits with an HND in Printing Management with Production. After leaving college she worked for a succession of large printing organisations as an Account Executive and a Print/Packaging estimator looking after blue chip accounts. It was only later through volunteering and working as a Supported Learning Tutor with a literacy project 2001-2004 that Davina became interested in Community Learning. A desire to learn more about working with communities lead her to study for the Bachelor of Community Learning and Development Degree at the University of Glasgow from 2004 – 2006. In January 2006 during her final year at University Davina secured a part time position with PPRC coordinating the Community Voices project. In November of the same year the position became full-time. Davina values the freedom to act that being part of the CAT gives her.

Hazel Lindsay

Hazel was born and raised in Drumchapel, Glasgow. She was brought up by her Mum and Gran in an environment where community activism and learning throughout life were part of who they were. From a very early age she has been active in communities on a voluntary basis working with people in a variety of settings from Women's Groups to Citizens Advice Bureau Debt Advice. All with the ultimate aims of empowerment, improving lives, making changes and escaping poverty. Hazel currently works in the field of Community Learning and Development as an Adult Literacies Development Worker working with people with Additional Learning Support Needs. She also remain active in my local community and find the voluntary work satisfying as it enables her to challenge oppressive attitudes and behaviours with more freedom. Hazel is a Community Councillor in her local area and actively enjoys giving back to the community that enriched her with life experiences.

Sara Jane McNeil

Sarah Jane McNeil is the Youth Development Worker at the Volunteer Centre Inverclyde, which is a project of Inverclyde Community Development Trust. She is a Graduate of the University of Glasgow, gaining her BA in Community Development with Merit. Her background is in Youth Work but has currently developed and facilitated a training programme for Volunteers of all ages and backgrounds. Her interests lie in Women's Studies and Theatre for Social Change

Lisa Peet

Lisa trained and worked as a youth worker for many years in the city of Nottingham, after discovering her passion for young people and holistic issues regarding the plain fact of being young. She then worked for a few years with homeless pregnant teenage girls and women at one of Framework Housing Associations hostels. Lisa then decided to relocate to Scotland and settled in Ayrshire working in children's homes and moving onto working as a 'through care' worker to assist with their transitions into adulthood. These experiences enabled her to see the society from a community development perspective. She furthered this education by attending Glasgow University to put it all into perspective and gained a BA in Community Development.

Janice Quinn

Janice Quinn was born and brought up in the East End of Glasgow, the second youngest in a family of seven. She was always aware of the impact poverty and the lack of opportunity had on the local community. She worked in a variety of different employment, and after the birth of her daughter established her own business working from home. The untimely death of her brother prompted her to reflect on her life and her contribution to those in need. She began volunteering, serving food to the homeless who walked the streets of the East End, and then went on to work for HOPE who encouraged her to pursue a degree in Community Development. She continues to work for HOPE and is in her fifth year as Coordinator of its Family & Addictions Project

Rosemary Robertson

Rosemary Robertson is a 33 year old mum to 10 year old Ross. Born in the East End of Glasgow, Rosie continues to live and work there as a Community Learning Co-ordinator. Having experienced community development as volunteer, adult learner, and worker she is delighted to have achieved a BA in Community Development at the University of Glasgow. Rosie recognises the support she received from PEEPS (Parents of East End Primary Schools) and their partners as having been a major contributing factor to her success. She expresses gratitude and love for all at PEEPS, Lesley, her friend and mentor whose humour made the pressure of study seem less, and her mum and son for providing her with the patience, love and understanding she needed to cope with the demands of study and work. Rosie describes the community centre where she completed her placement as *"a wonderful organisation who allowed me to me learn from them and attempt to put theory into practice"* and is thankful for the experience and relationships she gained there. Rosie intends to use what she has learned in her own community and hopes that her success will help her to support others who currently face some of the barriers to learning that she once experienced before becoming involved with PEEPS.

Trishna Sing

Trishna is a highly motivated and experienced Community Development Worker in the voluntary sector with the BME community. She was born in Oatlands Glasgow 1953 and went to Wolseley Street Primary, Mellville Street and then onto Kinning Park secondary school at 13. Trisha lived at home until her marriage in 1974 when she moved to Edinburgh. She started work as community development worker in 1989 with Sikh Sanjog and have remained with the organisation throughout. Trishna obtained her Degree in Community Learning and Development in 2007 from Glasgow University, and says this was her greatest achievement.

Lesley Ward

Lesley is a 42 year old mum of 3 boys, Jamie, Mark and Kieran and lives in Glasgow's East end with her partner Dave. Lesley is a firm believer in peer education and without the support from her fellow students, especially Rosie; she believes she would not have gotten through the past 3 years and reach her goal of achieving a BA in Community Development. A community development worker, Lesley is employed by an adult learning project and promotes the benefits of community involvement for the community in which she lives and works. Lesley was brought up in Drumchapel, Glasgow, where she first experienced the camaraderie of community and the sense of belonging it provided. She would like to say a huge thank you to Dave, who by all accounts should now be able to apply for jobs in community work!

The Context Of Contemporary Practice

> The only freedom supposed to be left to the masses is that of grazing on the ration of simulacra the system distributes to each individual.
>
> Michel de Certeau

This chapter explores two key questions about contemporary community development practice:

- What does community development achieve?
- Given we are where we are, is there is a need for a reinvented praxis informed by alternative theoretical perspectives?

Introduction

The dominant trend in UK social policy throughout the 20th century and onto today has been for the state to impose a modernist meta-narrative of increasing control on ever expanding areas of daily life. For good and not so good reasons the state now operates routine surveillance on our work and leisure activity through CCTV, scans emails and txt messages for potentially threatening content, and intervenes in what was once private and domestic life. Of course this is beneficial if it prevents domestic abuse, increases child protection, and reduces incidents of racial harassment. On the other hand some of this is simply bureaucratic interference in our daily life and more significantly alters the power balance between the citizen and the state. Underpinning these developments is the growing influence of communitarian thought that tells us that we have too many rights (which by implication we abuse) and do not take enough responsibility for ourselves, our family and our 'community'.

In the last 20 years or thereabouts community development has been seen by the state, albeit in a rather haphazard way, as a vehicle to promote aspects of this policy agenda. Although the language used in policy documents is often of local control and empowerment, the actual work has been based on pre-defined objectives, targets, milestones, and so on where the community development process is simply a means to an end. That end being to lock community activity, and potentially troublesome community activists, into the objectives and processes of the local state.

This would not be so bad if the dominant ideology of partnerships led to significant changes the quality of life and general wellbeing of the people concerned. Although individual successes can always be identified, this inherent managerialist model of practice fails overall. Burkett comments:

> *"In a complex world perhaps the most important questions regarding community development are those which seek to engage with human complexity, difference and mystery. They are not questions that will be solved by technical rationality – they are questions that are both deeply personal and deeply reflective of the social realities of the twenty first century"* (Burkett, 2001: 244)

Burkett's statement suggests that we need to develop new ways of working, to rediscover ways of working we have abandoned due to the requirements of partnership engagement, and equip ourselves with different theoretical perspectives to inform and direct our practice. Such an approach needs to better reflect the current postmodern condition and prioritises an open and reflective process that goes where the people concerned what it to go

What does community development achieve?

We could spend a long time debating the purpose of community development. To cut this short it is appropriate to defer to the National Occupational Standards for Community Development. These standards have recently been revised. At the time of writing the revised standards have not been formally released by the LLUK Standards Council but the final version of the revision states the key purpose of community development in the following terms:

> *Community Development is a long–term value based process which aims to address imbalances in power and bring about change founded on social justice, equality and inclusion.*
>
> *The process enables people to organise and work together to:*
>
> - *identify their own needs and aspirations*
> - *take action to exert influence on the decisions which affect their lives,*
>
> *improve the quality of their own lives, the communities in which they live, and societies of which they are a part.*

This view is partly a historical legacy statement which reflects one of the roots of community development in community action and protest movements. However, any substantial overview of community development in the UK today would be hard pressed to honestly identify the majority of practice as effectively tackling the structural issues and inequalities implied in the above statement. It is true that at the micro level social justice issues, equality and inclusion work is undertaken; but we have to ask to what real long term effect? A second question is how far do the local people involved in community development actually identify their own needs and aspirations, or do people in the main work on the agendas of local agencies.

As my colleague Dave Beck and I have suggested elsewhere (Beck and Purcell 2010) there is much rhetoric in social policy documents on the benefits of partnership working. It is argued that the incorporation of community development practice and local community groups and organisations into the partnership structures can at times be an effective mechanism for empowerment. There is no doubt that useful work gets done, but what are the opportunity costs from over reliance on the partnership model?

As suggested above our alternative view is that partnership working is one of a number of mechanisms of social policy which function to extend institutional and bureaucratic control over people's lives. Partnerships generally identify local needs through statistical analysis. Hot spots of need are by some magic sweep of a planner's pen on map defined in terms of community. Often these communities only exist in the mind of social planners and do not reflect the actual relationships and networks of people who live there. Either way the process tends to make the identified social issue a problem for local people to solve.

Agencies develop projects and targets, and community development workers go forth to recruit local people or existing community groups to work on this agenda. Partly this is a contemporary social policy objective of modern societies. It is also one of the consequences of what is called managerialism. In effect it has reduced what should be a dynamic and creative process driven by local people expressing and responding to real local issues and needs, to one of top down bureaucratisation.

Like any social practice community development today is inevitably a product of historical development and the policy maker's own ideological position. It is worth summarising how we got to where we are now.

Community development has number of roots in evolving to its current form. One strand is of radical protest which as we have noted appears to be in decline. Depending upon how you read social history this could be traced back to the 19th century Chartists, the Suffragettes, the Jarrow March, through post war housing campaigns to current environmental protests around road and airports to name but a few. The other and more dominant strand is the steady movement of establishing development work with poor and disadvantaged people as a profession alongside the creation of social work.

This dominant strand can be linked to the creation of urban settlements in the new industrial 19th century cities. The motivation for this development came from the philanthropic middle classes who were concerned at the social costs and effects of industrialisation on the poorer elements of the working class. The settlements were concerned with welfare and self improvement through education. Inevitably this meant that the responsibility for improvement was placed on the individual. Even though it was accepted that economic change was the driver for many of the social problems, there was no question of a structural analysis of this or any campaigns for radical change.

From the late 1930's onwards and especially in the immediate post war period the idea of supporting ideals of community took off. Various government ministries produced policy positions aimed to assist people to settle into new towns and estates and live a normative life around work, educational and leisure activities. To promote these objectives officials were recruited to work on local housing estates. Many of these workers had experience in the colonies of the British Empire, where embryonic ideas of community development had been created to facilitate the integration of local people into colonial systems of administration.

The watershed on the road to establishing community development as a respected professional activity for the state was the Gulbenkian Foundation report in 1968 on 'Community Work and Social Change'. The report was influenced by social policy in the USA which focused on integrating black neighbourhoods into the social mainstream. The Gulbenkian Report identified three main activities for community work: the democratic process of involving people in services that affect their lives, personal fulfilment of belonging to a community, and as aid to community planning. In particular these activities should take place in what was then called 'twilight areas' and new communities. It is a short road from Gulbenkian to the current domination by local partnerships.

The next step on the road was the establishment, also in 1968 of the Community Development Projects by the Home Office. Although triggered by what was then called the 'rediscovery of poverty' across the UK, the CDP's were concentrated in very small and localised areas and tasked with co-ordinating local state activities and linking in local citizens to that process. To their credit some of the CDP's recognised that the causes of poverty then (as they are now) are economic and structural and that local area working is essentially applying sticking plaster to a broken leg (see CDP 1977a, 1977b).

From the CDP's three models of practice were developed. Firstly 'amelioration' based on practical responses to poverty based around self help. Secondly, what has been termed the 'traditional response' that sought to increase local community control over the allocation of resources to deprived areas. And thirdly, a 'radical response' that tried to develop a class analysis and build national coalitions, including trade unions, to tackle structural issues. Perhaps because it avoids any serious ideological debate or challenge to the status quo, the amelioration strand has come to be the most prevalent of the three models.

Through the 1980's and 1990's all these approaches began to respond to the increasingly influential feminist movement and Black perspectives work. This led slowly to a movement away from a mainly white male working class position which had dominated community development thinking and practice. By the year 2000 community development workers tended to equip themselves with a value set which reflected perspective around gender, race, sexuality and ethnicity. However, the practice on the ground continues to be localised and focused mainly on a mixture self help and linking people into local planning processes. Since the election of New Labour in 1997 community development has increasingly been built into the social inclusion strategy of the government. The route for local change is through consensual partnership working with key interface roles for community development.

The classic community work text book of last 15 years or so, Skills in Neighbourhood Work (Henderson and Thomas 1992, reprinted 2002) reduced practice to a series of steps around entering a community, identifying localised needs, settings goals, forming and building organisations, dealing with decision makers and leaving once the objective had been achieved. In sense the book is a very practical guide on how to do mainstream practice. However, by identifying the omissions in the book (e.g. explicit discussion of ideology and theories) we can learn a lot about the position and purpose of community development practice from the establishment perspective.

In contrast this managerial and skills based approach to practice there is the postmodern argument that our lives are now subject to ever increasing control. Community development practice should be about responding to people and local organisations as autonomous individuals capable of deciding their own future. Partnerships it could be argued despite the rhetoric, simply treat people, organisations as communities as objects to be analysed, categorised and organised to pre determined ends. Beck and Purcell argue that the partnership approach has inbuilt deficiencies as a practice model. Specifically it:

- Ignores the wider effects of globalisation, structural inequality etc,

- Ignores the debates around feminism, identity, culture, sexuality, etc.
- Is weak on exploring the values underpinning practice
- Fails to adopt a rights driven perspective
- Promotes models of participation where local people are largely powerless
- Draws people into establishment planning structures at the expense of developing local autonomous and powerful organisations
- Light on any underpinning theory
- Accepts the political status quo (Normative, Communitarian)
- Based on an ideal of a mythical community
- Does not reach the approximately 2.5% of the population (sometimes called the 'unreachables') who are in most need.

Part of the current problem for community development is the very loose and undefined use of the term community. Planners happily draw lines on maps and designate everyone inside it as being members of a community. Such a view is based upon the now orthodoxy derived from the Chicago School of Sociology and the work of Robert Park. Inherent in their view was that simply living near someone meant that you would have similar needs and interests. Consequently, people would act together to make the supposed community work better. This can happen at times of major stress or threat. For example the proposed building of an open cast coal mine next to a housing estate.

However, it is usually not like that. The following research study from Beck and Purcell illustrates the point.

> The focus of the study was to explore the effect on a small town that was in the process of expansion through the construction of new private housing estates. The concern of the local authority was that the 'community' developing in the new estates would not integrate with the existing 'community' of the old town.
>
> The old town had developed around the local coal mining industry which no longer exists. The Miners Welfare Hall provided a focus to the area and organised the local gala; the

main social event of the year. Research showed that a significant minority of the local population were involved with the Miners Welfare in some way over the year.

There was no evidence that the old town had a single overarching community in any way. The research team identified many micro communities. Usually these were based on extended family networks and relationships developed from school. These micro communities tended to overlap in membership. However, this overlap was not sufficient to link everyone living in the local area together. Attitudes to the old town and desires for the future were varied; it was not possible to identify any commonalities or desires or concerns across the old town population.

The new estates mostly housed people who had moved from the nearby major city. They tended to work in the city, shop at out of town malls, have family and friends dispersed across the region. In effect many people on the new estates lived their lives across a wide geographical area. Contact with the old town and the existing population there was limited and mainly focused on the primary school. There was little evidence that people on the new estates interacted significantly with each other.

The local authority wanted a formula that would enable them to understand how many new houses they could build before it became too difficult for the new community to integrate with the old community. The answer to their question was that not only was the new estates not a community in any functional sense, the old town was not a single community either. Integration, although a desirable policy goal, would not happen as there were not sufficient common interests and activities for this to happen

One of the best analyses of what community means and how they function comes from the anthropologist Anthony Cohen. He argues that community is not created by the structure of the housing estate or village. The simple fact of people living in proximity to each other does not make a community. Instead community is a cultural belief in the minds of people. Or as Cohen put it "*community exists in the minds of its members, and should not be confused with geographical or sociographic assertions of fact*" (2003).

I feel myself to be part of a community built around the local football team where I lived as a teenager. Even though that was in London and I now live in Glasgow, I still feel and act as part of that community. The housing estate where I currently live has lots of micro communities. For example there are several groups of young people who wander around the estate at night, there are various men from different part of the estate who meet up in the local pub, there are groups of women who have children of the same age and who meet at nursery or at the school. Other local people know each other from working for the same company. However, like the example cited above there is no over arching community in any operational sense. Like many of the residents in the new estate above I am not part of any of the local micro communities as my life pattern is diffused over a very wide geographical area.

There is a very close relationship between the proliferation of micro communities and the ideas of social capital. A key task of community workers is to build social capital; that is to enhance the *bonds* between people who have shared interests and characteristics, to make *bridging* relationship between people of different social groups, *link* people across social classes and power differentials, to build *trust* between people based on *reciprocity* of actions. Robert Putnam (2001) argues that where social capital is high people:

- Feel they are part of various communities
- Will participate in local networks and organisations
- Will help others in time of need
- Will welcome strangers
- Will help out with something (but no one will do everything)

However, the areas in which most community development workers operate have as a consequence of poverty and inequality low social capital. To enhance social capital community development workers need to build from existing micro communities.

The need for reinvented praxis: some theoretical perspectives

Most community development workers would say they have a value position, although from the practice studies it is not always clear how much this influences practice across the board. Fewer workers would be able to provide an underpinning theoretical position for what they do. This is a critical question: is community development just a process for organising local activity or is it a practical application of a theoretical understanding of society and social change?

We argue it has to be the latter. One of the questions that need further exploration is what we actually mean by change. There are a number of perspectives here:

- **Individual change** in terms of skills, knowledge and as Freire said building confidence for people to move their 'boundary situations'.
- **Economic change** to equalise distribution of wealth, reduce inequality and poverty.
- **The promotion of social justice** to challenge oppression powerlessness and promote civil liberties and human rights.

For those who take this view much attention is given to the work of Freire and Gramsci and general theories around social change and social movements. It can be argued that this in itself is not sufficient and we could useful explore what are called 'theories of everyday life'. This section provides a summary of these ideas.

The starting point therefore is with Freire and Gramsci. Both Gramsci and Freire come from a Marxist tradition so have an underlying common analysis that leads to many similarities in ideas. However, Gramsci was thinking about a western European society in the 1930's, whereas Freire was writing about developing countries in the 1970/80's. Marxism and social theory in general had changed significantly since Gramsci's time, so there are also differences in his ideas. The following analysis is based partially on the work of Peter Mayo (1999) and Brookfield (1987) and the authors own interpretation.

The positions outlined in the similarities section provide us with a framework from which to analyse practice, and contextualises the context within which practices takes place. The section on differences poses questions about the nature of society and can usefully be explored to increase our understanding, and help us to develop personal positions on these questions.

Similarities:

- All education is political, being based upon an ideological position
- The ruling order will use coercion if necessary to sustain their power
- Civil society is an area of social and ideological conflict where cultural / educational process need to change from dominant to transformational / counter hegemonic discourse
- Strong belief in the ability of people to organise and create change
- Intellectuals / educators are also part of a process and need to learn from it, rather than experts who simply control it
- The role of adult educators (and related workers) is to facilitate the challenging of the notion of normative 'common sense' and the everyday acceptance of how things are as being both right and inevitable.
- People should move from being *objects* that are controlled by institutions to *subjects* in control of their own destiny
- The importance of Praxis (linking knowledge to theory to action)
- Transformation through education will be most effective if linked to mass organisations and social movements
- Local collective education; Gramsci through factory councils, Freire through cultural circles.

Differences:

- Gramsci was concerned essentially with the traditional Marxist concept of the working class. Freire and broader Freirean practice identifies multiple sites of engagement around gender, sexuality, race and identity issues as well as the economic.
- Freire was influenced by the ideas of poststructuralists. They believed that we all develop our own individual interpretation of who we are and how we fit in a subjective analysis of society

- Gramsci was interested in the conflicts between high (establishment) and low (working class culture). Freire is almost entirely concerned with exploring what he terms popular culture.
- Gramsci wanted a critical interpretation of history so the working class could understand the context of present society. Freire is mostly concerned with understanding the present and places less importance on the past.
- Freire believed that traditional teacher led education (banking education) filled the student like an empty vessel. Gramsci thought that education was filtered by the individual's experiences and that all teaching was reinterpreted by the learner.
- Models of Freirean practice are well established, whereas Gramscian practice is more about intent and perspective than defined ways of working.

Freire and Gramsci are clearly very helpful in providing community development workers with a theoretical underpinning to practice. However, it may be that we need more than this. For example we could learn a lot from the counter cultural writings of Ivan Illich, and what could be called the discourse around the nature of 'everyday life' and look at the work of Henri Lefebvre and Michel de Certeau.

Ivan Illich (1990, 1997) asks a fundamental question on what development work is for; is it about increased consumption of goods and services or for an improved quality of life? If the latter, how can this be defined in non materialistic and sustainable ways? Illich (2005) also questions both the effectiveness and purpose of our modern institutions (education, social work, policing, and health). He believed that large organisations inevitably operate in their own interest and that development and the tackling of social needs can only be defined in terms of more of the same. If the community is not safe we need more police, if people are unhealthy we need more hospitals, if children fail to perform in school we need more teachers, and so on. What is seldom asked, suggests Illich is how people can change these things for themselves through re-visioning their lives and building new forms of association.

Henri Lefebvre (2008) starts from the position that the real nature of everyday life is not as it appears to be. We live in a hegemonic society where we have learned a common sense view of right and wrong and know that we need to conform to authority. Daily life takes places in the organised spaces of the modern world; in workplaces, on commuter trains, in leisure places (pubs, cinemas, parks, community centres) and so on. However, our implicit acceptance of what is, and our conformity of how to behave in designated spaces is nothing more than obedience to socially constructed norms, which in turn are based on manifestations of the dominant ideology and power relationships.

de Certeau (1984) explores how experience of everyday life is controlled by the institutions (corporations, local state, public services, police, etc) through their control of space. He termed these dominant activities *strategies*. These strategies operate in various ways through private security patrolling shopping malls, through the informal signs that tell various sub groups that particular spaces are not for them, to redesigning urban building and open areas to prevent people from simply sitting around, to how community centres are run and lettings policies.

For de Certeau the effect of this overarching web of control was to create an alienated life. As individuals we have a desire to make life more liveable and try often unconsciously to subvert the rules and attempts at social control, to make our life a bit more liveable. De Certeau called these responses *tactics*. Mostly, tactics are individualised, sometimes positive, sometimes anti social, often trivial gestures. For example, walking where you are not supposed to be, taking extra time for lunch, playing on Facebook in work time, downloading software without paying for it, using work stationary at home, and so on.

In this context it is easy to blame others for your situation and see little to be gained from engaging in community activity. When we do enter into collective action it tends to be through what Guy Debord termed the '*spectacle*'. Instead of actively campaigning on third world debt, or make serious changes to our lifestyle, we just buy and consume a protest. We buy the armband, attend the benefit concert, buy the charity CD, and generally live our lives through selected media interpretations of experience.

The challenge for community development is to help people rethink what they want to do with their lives. As Freire argues to move from a naïve view of the world that lacks reflection and analysis to one of critical consciousness where there is sufficient understanding to enable change to take place. In Freirean practice this involves facilitating people through a Reflection – Vision – Planning – Action cycle. The key to success is in effectively helping people in the reflection – vision stage. To do this we need not only to unpack our experience of life to date and to better understand how the world operates; we also need further tools to help us think about how the world might be.

Towards a new paradigm of practice

Part of the problem we face is that the nature and quality of life is defined in terms of money. We work to earn money and our social life is predicated on spending it; shopping as leisure, relationships defined through gifts, and as discussed above political action through purchasing the right products. One of the themes of a contemporary postmodernist analysis of society is that people are seen to be defined by what they consume. We judge others through the clothes they wear, the car they drive, their mobile phone. We construct our own identity through a similar process of consumption. In this context building community and collective action becomes somewhat irrelevant.

We need to remember Maslow's hierarchy (1943) which shows us that whereas the basic levels of human need (physiological and safety) generally require the spending of money. The higher levels are based on the quality of relationships, stock of social capital and self perception. Trying to meet these needs through consumerism is what we tend to do, but this does not work. A range of studies show that happiness is based on a range of cultural factors rather than simply how much money you have. See for example the box at the end of the chapter reporting on the Plateau of Happiness that tries to map the degree of happiness in a country against income. For a development of this argument see the papers from the Rethinking Development Conference (http://www.gpiatlantic.org/conference/).

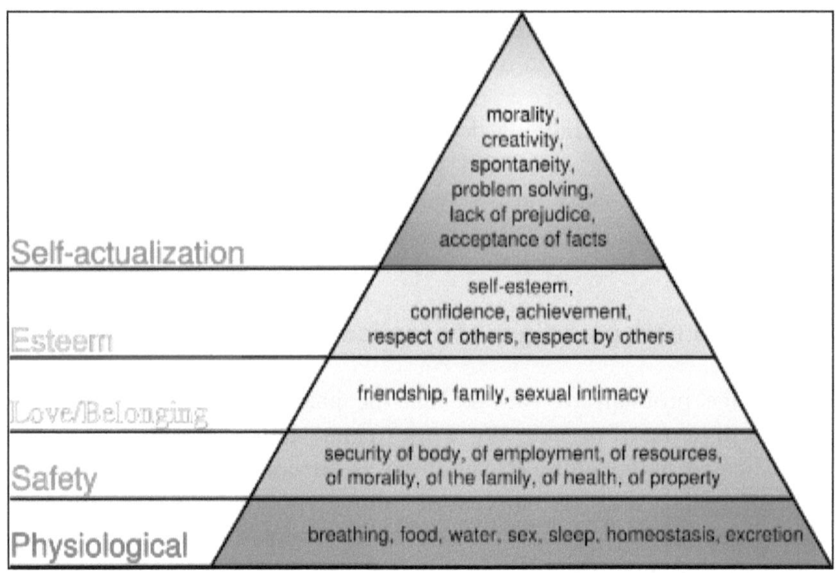

This is not to suggest that we should incorporate happiness into some managerial framework that defines it, sets happiness targets and milestones and re-designates community development staff as Happiness Agents. This would miss the point. Rather we are suggesting social policy should take the improvement of happiness as a goal, and we should explore with people in the reflection – vision phase of the work what makes them happy, and look for practical ways to assist people to make their lives happier.

As de Certeau might have said we should develop tactics for happiness. It might be thought that this was obvious. But looking at people being organised into constituted groups, battling for funding, populating partnership sub groups and meeting in depressing buildings on cold nights to refine local policy, this can often not be the case.

This is not to suggest that involvement in community development is a joyful ride. A process of critical reflection on your life may lead to doubts, conflicts, sad memories and periods of unhappiness. In the medium term though, an effective community development process should lead to increased personal confidence, a greater knowledge of self, improved self esteem, a greater range of social contacts and a higher stock of social capital. Taken together such process of change should increase happiness.

Happiness though is a difficult concept to pin down. Work has been done here, but more progress has been made on an associated and overlapping concept of wellbeing. Academics, as they are prone to do, have developed metrics to try and suggest how wellness as a contributor to happiness as a concept might be measured. One example was to use 7 measures (Jones 2006):

1. **Economic Wellness**: consumer debt, average income to consumer price index ratio and income distribution
2. **Environmental Wellness**: pollution, noise and traffic
3. **Physical Wellness**: measurement of physical health metrics such as severe illnesses
4. **Mental Wellness**: usage of antidepressants and rise or decline of psychotherapy patients
5. **Workplace Wellness**: job change, workplace complaints and lawsuits
6. **Social Wellness**: discrimination, safety, divorce rates, complaints of domestic conflicts and family lawsuits, public lawsuits, crime rates
7. **Political Wellness**: quality of local democracy, individual freedom, and foreign conflicts.

The New Economics Foundation (IACD 2009) suggests that wellbeing has to be understood in the context of our local ecosystem. NEF argue that:

- Human wellbeing is based upon the nature and interaction of culture, education, social capital, governance, healthcare and economy
- Ecosystem wellbeing is based upon the nature and interaction of natural capital, water quality, biodiversity, CO2 omissions, air quality and soil erosion

The critical factors here will vary according to setting, but all these factors are important. Just because those of us who live in developed economies take many of the ecosystem factors for granted does not diminish their importance.

The Satisfaction with Life Index takes a different approach and attempt to rank the subjective satisfaction with life across 178 countries. The UK ranks at 41 behind Bhutan (who we will come to shortly) at 8, Costa Rica at 13 and Dominica at 29. These and several other countries above us in the ranking have a significantly lower GDP to that of the UK.

In Bhutan the government has decide to introduce a national indicator and policy driver called Gross National Happiness (GNH). Writing on GNH Tshoki Zangmo comments that:

> *Research studies around the world have shown that although economic growth has increased steeply over the past decades, there has been no rise in well-being. GNH stands for holistic approach towards governance as it values not only the economic capital but also the social, emotional and spiritual needs of the people.*
>
> *A GNH society calls for the inclusion of people's perceptions on their well-being. The domain of psychological well-being consists of the outcomes of life circumstances and achievements. For these reasons we should measure this valued outcome so that policy makers are better informed and situations are better assessed. It is essential for policy decisions to be influenced by issues related to psychological well-being. Psychological well-being indicators attempt to understand people's evaluations of their lives.*
>
> *Currently, we have four broad categories under which we attempt to study psychological well-being of the Bhutanese people. They are life satisfaction, emotional well-being, spirituality, and stress. The findings of this research paper provide interesting policy-related issues but further continuous assessment of well-being would offer policy makers a much stronger basis to making informed policy decisions. Our proposed system of psychological well-being indicators is aimed to not only supplement economic indicators but also to enhance their value by placing them within overall framework of tracking GNH.*

Surveys in Bhutan indicate that the top five criteria for a happy life are, in the order of importance;

1. Financial security
2. Transportation
3. Education
4. Good health
5. Family relationships

For each country the ranking of factors is likely to vary and it would be interesting to pose the question of the top five factors for being happy within the communities where we work.

These studies provide us with food for thought. Whilst not advocating creating metrics like this, the above categories do give us useful headings to explore. In terms of Freirean practice each of these headings could be explored as generative themes. In doing so we could refocus community development work to activities that consciously and creatively worked to improve happiness and wellbeing as defined by the local people themselves and recognise that the mix of concerns and ambitions would vary. Perhaps we could re-evaluate what we do. Some of our current practice will promote happiness, a lot of it would probably claim that it does but probably fails to do so, and some of our work may be if we are honest actually pointless or actively creating unhappiness. We ought to know!

The next section of the book explores the case studies, and they could be read with the above discussion in mind.

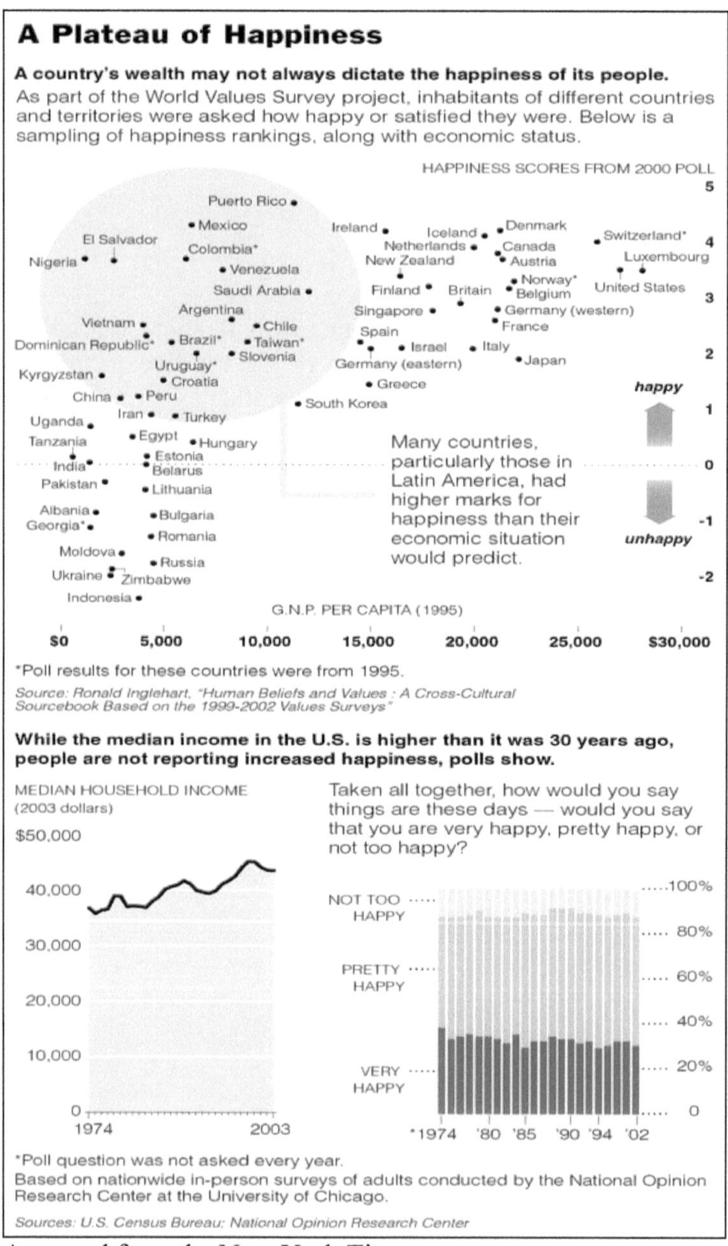

Accessed from the New York Times http://www.nytimes.com/imagepages/2005/10/03/science/20051004_HAPP_GRAPHIC.html

The Practice Studies

Leadership does not depend on being right.

Ivan Illich

Practice Study 1

Community Initiative to Reduce Violence

Lesley Ward

Abstract

This practice study looks at some of the issues around inner city gangs. It is based with a Police initiative and explores the potential of working with parents of those involved in gang activity. The study focuses on establishing a parent support group. The merits of doing this are discussed.

The Study

This work was undertaken with the Community Initiative to Reduce Violence (CIRV) The main aim was to assist communities to plan and take collective action and to support communities to monitor actions and review action for change.

CIRV is a multi-agency partnership and community based initiative, headed by Strathclyde Police, designed to reduce violent behaviour amongst violent gang members in Glasgow focused on the East End of Glasgow. The fundamental aims of CIRV is to achieve this reduction of street gang violence by targeting specific areas, to quickly and dramatically reduce weapon related violence, with sustained reductions over time.

CIRV also aims to deliver a clear message to violent street gangs;: the violence must stop. This message is communicated through a number of different mechanisms, including self referral call-in sessions, direct contact through street workers, police, prisons, school campus officers, community outreach workers and, when the time is right, the media. A full range of alternatives to chaotic gang lifestyles are made available to those choosing to engage and will include education, employment, diversion, change programmes and support services.

At a meeting with the Community Team lead worker it became clear that there was an underlying perception that most gang members were children who come from one parent or dysfunctional families. This is a common perception which is often promoted by the media and believed by the public, and it seems, those members of the public who are paid to serve communities. I am of the opinion that young people who find themselves in trouble with the police are at a disadvantage from the outset.

Further meetings were set up with the manager to discuss possible options. They realised that for the initiative to be sustainable one of the fundamental aims would be to enlist the support of parents of gang members, who in turn would support their sons' involvement with them. The plan was for me to work with a group of parents whose children have engaged with CIRV. I was informed at this stage that these parents had already identified the need for a support group and all that remained to do was to arrange a venue and date for an information session. However, this was not the case and I found that a lot of my placement time was spent writing letters and making phone calls to parents of boys on the CIRV data base.

I felt excited about working with this group as I have extensive personal first hand experience of the gang culture and how families can be drastically affected. I thought as I could empathise with these parents it would set me in good standing in gaining trust within the group. It is my experience that people warm to you more if you understand what they are experiencing.

However, I was keen to make the group aware that I did not have all the answers, what I experienced and how I dealt with my own situation may not suit everyone. Anne Hope and Sally Timmel in Training for Transformation (2007) speak of Paulo Freire and his theory of banking education, where "*the teacher makes regular deposits in the empty mind of the pupil"* (2007: 17). It was imperative to this group and any other group that they do not rely on one person to provide information and solely rely on this to be correct. As my training is in adult education I am a firm believer in peer education where learners learn from each other and also where the teacher learns from the learner.

On reflection, I chose this project as I wanted to imbed myself within an organisation such as the head of the initiative (Strathclyde Police) which in my opinion has a top down approach to working with communities. I was aware that I may have been putting myself in a situation where my values as a community worker may conflict with those of the initiative, but I was interested whether I would be strong enough to constructively challenge those in power if this transpired.

My role would be to support the group, to assist them to engage with each other and to find ways of increasing group numbers. I would also explain the mechanisms of groups; discuss group aims and objectives and roles which can exist within groups. I would support them with agreed action plans and help them to achieve goals for their group and on an individual basis. I would report back to CIRV with a report on progress after each meeting

On my first day of direct work I contacted the parents of boys who are actively engaging with CIRV. The idea was that these parents, whilst being supported within a group, would be able to support their sons whilst participating in activities. Although this sounded logical, I felt that this was not being inclusive to people in communities whose children are not involved with CIRV or those whose boys were not complying with CIRV aims and objectives. This was a contradiction to the way I would have chosen to engage with people and this made me feel unsure about my role. Surely the parents of boys involved in gangs but not yet engaged with CIRV were the ones who would need more support? I knew I would have to become more vocal with my opinions if I was to stand a chance of supporting the parents form their group. I was not happy that I may be guilty of bringing a group of parents together not to support each other but to strengthen the CIRV initiative.

In relation to the values of community development work I strongly believe that everyone has a right to fully participate in decision- making processes that can affect their lives, so by being selective in contacting parents I was going directly against these values which I relate to in my practice.

Together with developing a group I was also learning to fit in with the CIRV team which was also a group, this was a fantastic learning curve for me giving me an ideal opportunity to enter into the process of Bruce Tuckman's team development model. Tuckman (1965) believes groups experience 4 stages of group development; forming – storming - norming and performing.

Working closely with the CIRV admin assistant to obtain client information I took the lead role in contacting parents personally in advance of sending formal written invitations which were professionally prepared and outlined the concept of the Parent Support Group.

I arranged and catered a meeting within a local community facility which was selected for ease of access and in a relaxed and comfortable environment. I advised parents that a detailed presentation would be shown at the initial meeting. I developed this presentation along with the CIRV Team Leader.

5 people came to the initial meeting. I felt this was a good response as only 12 parents were contacted. On the night of the meeting I decided that the presentation would be too formal and we decided to just talk about the initiative and what it was providing for their sons. I felt that the meeting was overloaded with CIRV aims and not enough time was left for the important support message. My project co-worker led most of the meeting and I am sure it was as he is as passionate about supporting the gang members as I am about supporting parents.

On reflection I should have remained with the power point presentation as this would have given structure to the presentation and provided me with an equal amount of time to speak with the parents. However, good discussions were held at this meeting and progress was already in the early stages.

We know from Henderson and Thomas that *'people will become engaged with community groups for a number of reasons: to improve the quality of life within their community, and too protect their personal and /or family interests'* (2002: 217). These were the reasons people joined this group. In working and learning together the group were clearly able to see the benefits of sharing experiences and how this could assist them to overcome problems relating to their families. The group admitted that this was the first time they were able to speak with people in the same situation and that they felt valued as an individual due to the amount of knowledge they brought to the table. They openly admitted how their sons' behaviour deeply affected others within their community and felt a degree of shame but also anger as they are often the target of gossip.

One group member related indirectly to conflict within communities. She shared with the group that she had previously tried to take direct action and organise a meeting between mothers of boys who were in gangs. One street in her community was split in half by rival gangs and she felt if all the mothers got together then the rivalry may be able to be dealt with. It was not successful and to date the street is still affected by gang violence. Her hope would be to try involving these parents again with the possibility of inviting them to join the group.

Margaret Ledwith suggests that *"little stories" restore self-respect through dignity, mutuality and conviviality"* (2005: 65). So at the second meeting I invited the parents to say why they came along to the group. The parents were forthcoming in their stories and how they came to be in their situation. Supporting them through this process by ensuring they did not speak too personally so early on in the formation of the group I encouraged them to delve a little deeper into their own experiences of childhood and the roles their parents played in their lives. By being reflexive, they were able to see historical links to their boys' involvement with gangs. Ledwith goes on to say, *"by reaching inside themselves and their histories, she uses this approach with her students to develop reflection and story as a discovery of who they are and what has shaped them in their world"* (2005: 65) Ledwith describes this process as *critical consciousness.* Although the group touched on this in this session I am aware that they are a degree away from relating their experiences with that of local/ global context, however, I would say they began to form links to the wider community by listening to others in the group who shared similar stories.

At the third meeting I took the group through the process of creating an action plan and explaining the benefits of this. The group's main aims at this stage were;

1. To involve more parents
2. Publicise the group
3. Get training in basic IT skills.

As the group relied on me to encourage more parents to participate this task was given to me. The outcome of this was for me to discuss the possibility of contacting all parents on the CIRV data base with a written invite to attend. The response was one more parent joining and one enquiry. It was very obvious to me and the group that sending letters out to people was not an effective method to encourage participation. I felt that face to face contact was a more productive method of engaging with people although this was not an option due to the nature of the group.

Negatively speaking, this was not an ideal situation as the group were relying on me and the CIRV team to let others know about their group. The group were anxious to learn about computing for a few reasons. One of which was to learn how to access You Tube, a video sharing website where users can upload and share videos. They had heard their sons speak about this website and other parents had informed them they were able to track there sons' activities by accessing videos they appeared in. Indeed, this is one of the ways the police obtain gang information.

The group were keen to help each other and also help others in the community who are affected by the gang culture. Although at this stage the group had not thought of a way in which they could collectively bring about change for communities, they felt that by meeting every week they were beginning to change small things in their own lives which in turn may lead to bigger change.

In order for me to understand more clearly how the CIRV team worked it was decided that I should sit in on training sessions for Street Advocacy; these were employees of the Police, Education Department and Housing Department who would be in contact with gang members and their families. These street advocates would promote CIRV and encourage gang members to sign up to the initiative. Head gang members would be targeted and 'encouraged' to sign the CIRV pledge. It was clear from these training sessions if they did not comply then these gang members would be the target of the Police at every turn. Although I could see their reasons for working in this way, due to the level of violence on the streets in Glasgow's East End, I was troubled at the lack of social justice. This was in direct contrast to respecting civil and human rights, it was not in my opinion promoting a fairer society.

This led me to ask myself questions directed at CIRV:

- Was I brought in to fail? I feel that I was being used to prove that parents did not feel a need for a group and through the lack of support I was given, this may prove to be the case.
- Was an obvious gap identified and therefore *had* to be addressed?
- Was bringing me in a way to tick a box to prove they had tried to address this need but that it had failed to attract the parents in the way that was first hoped?

Whilst working with the team I saw little progress towards getting the clients into employment. The promises of jobs was spoken about strongly, although to date I have only heard of 10 clients securing a job. I sense that CIRV use this as a hook to persuade the gang members to engage with them, however in my opinion, most of these young men need considerable training prior to employment. CIRV workers are passionate about these young men to a degree; however, they are working for an organisation which has priorities which may not be as inclusive and socially accommodating as a community development approach. Stark differences were obvious between the police members and those such as social work and education where the latter took a more community development approach to working with the young men and their families.

In my reports to the CIRV team I was asked questions in relation to information that may have been shared about their clients through their parents. I made it clear I could not share any information, personal matters were strictly confidential. This was a ground rule that had been agreed with group. The CIRV team agreed in hindsight, apologising for any pressure they may have put on me to share information. Although I found this to be an uncomfortable situation I felt I dealt with it in the correct manner.

During my sessions with the group I took a structured and focussed approach. I encouraged the group to hold regular meetings within a community venue which I had secured for that purpose, the decision on how often the group met was left to them to decide. I advised the group of meeting protocols, agenda's etc and encouraged them to set S.M.A.R.T objectives, this is a process which helps to create specific, measureable, achievable, realistic and timed goals, and to develop an action plan which would outline their aims and objectives and agreed ownership/timescales. I allowed the group to debate at some length and come to an agreement on what was proposed.

Once again, I am in agreement with Henderson and Thomas who say, *"The importance of a worker helping a group turn their discontent into a series of needs, the needs into a range of objectives and the objectives into tasks and priorities is of crucial importance, not least because of the diversity of needs and problems that the people may experience"* (2002: 172). Although most of the aims and objectives were personal needs in the beginning, I encouraged the group to look at how these needs could be looked at collectively as a group as most of the needs were similar. We discussed ground rules and made a contract which the group agreed should be adhered to at all times.

The plan was I would support the group in the early stages and once they were comfortable with operating on their own I would leave. I would have to ensure the group were able to engage with the central CIRV co-ordination team for support when I was no longer there and so supplied them with the relevant communication channels which would effectively ensure contact was met. I assisted the group in developing Email contacts with each other to enhance inter group communication out with group meetings.

At an appropriate stage I introduced the group to the concepts of monitoring. I developed a focussed session plan which included interactive activity making the process easy to understand. The group had no previous knowledge of monitoring. However, I felt the way I explained monitoring simple terms, helping them to relate the process of monitoring in their personal lives and how they already do this without naming it, became a tool which they could see themselves using to their benefit.

We used the action plan to explore how we would know when we have achieved something, if it was achieved in the timescale etc. I also asked the group to think of times when they informally monitor, and gave an example of how they may monitor their sons' behaviour, how did they know something worked? And if not where did it go wrong?

I have introduced an action driven focus for change amongst the group who have become more organised as they develop. They are now clearly reviewing agreed actions on a regular basis and recording progress in the terms of minutes/ updated action plan for future review.

The parents have told me they rely on the weekly meetings to assist them through challenging times; most of the group have sons who remain involved in violent activities. If I have achieved one thing in this work it is that I have provided an opportunity where parents can have time on their own out with the chaotic lifestyle their sons present them with.

My role within the CIRV team was a considerable challenge; I came to CIRV with my own personal values, some of which I related directly to the values of Community Development Work. These equipped me with the strength to challenge structure within the initiative. After negotiations with the project manager a way forward was decided for this piece of work:

- A member of the CIRV team would be assigned the Parent Support Group as part of their role within the team, they would be the main contact and I would be the community support for as long as I remained to be a volunteer
- A new funding request for the group to be submitted to their main funders
- Group to be publicised on all CIRV promotional material
- Group to have space on the agenda at CIRV team meetings with a chance for the team to receive an update on progress and also for any group requests
- Any parents or family member in the community who feels the need for support due to their Childs activity in gangs or related violence will have access to the group.
- Support group to become a strand of CIRV

In conclusion I felt this was a huge achievement in terms of my role as a community development worker. I had the strength of conviction to fight for something the community felt there was a need for. I believe had I not met with the manager, the group would not have survived as they were viewed very much as a separate entity. Perhaps it was my own personal experience of gangs and how I felt there was a need for a support group which made me persist with my placement. I am unsure I would have been as committed without this. I found this work very challenging however, without these challenges I may not have developed as much in my practice.

Commentary

This study demonstrates a number of critical factors for successful practice.

Firstly, the worker has a very clear understanding of the underpinning values which keep community based work on track. This led to the worker questioning not only the various steps of the work (is it right to do this, and to do it this way), but also to skilfully confront some of the assumptions embedded within the CIRV.

Secondly, the worker clearly understands the process of engaging with people, establishing and maintaining a community based group. There are various theoretical models to assist workers with this process and she has made good use of both Henderson and Thomas and Tuckman.

It is important though to not get lost in the day to day work on the streets. The worker draws on ideas from Paulo Freire and a commentary on this by Ledwith to help her maintain a wider context and potential for the group work.

Finally, the worker is clearly operating in a reflexive mode. She is aware that she has personal experiences which influence her approach to the broad issues around gangs that influences how she thinks the work should progress, and realises that the way she presents herself has an impact on the group and other colleagues.

Questions are raised in the study about the nature of the partnerships implied in this work; between the police and other agencies, between the police and parents and other local residents. These questions are not followed through here but are fundamental to evaluating the potential and actual success of this type of work.

Practice Study 2

West Dunbartonshire Lesbian, Gay, Bisexual and Transgender Equality Network

Hazel Lindsay

Abstract

The practice study reports on the creation of a network for developing LGBT issues. Of particular note is that the work was developed from and supported by the local Community Planning Partnership. The study discusses organisational issues and outlines the work undertaken.

The Study

This case study looks at the initial stages of a newly established partnership, Lesbian, Gay, Bisexual and Transgender Equality Network (LGBTEN), in West Dunbartonshire. It looks at how and why the network was established, who was involved and what was achieved in its first year. It also includes an examination as to why there is a need to raise awareness of LGBT issues in West Dunbartonshire and how this fits with current policy and legislation as well as social attitudes and national agendas.

There is also an analysis of how the network partners functioned as a group in terms of taking on roles and responsibilities. This includes looking into the benefits and drawbacks of partnership working as well as how this contributed to any successes or pitfalls that it experienced.

A number of lessons were learned throughout the initial stages of the networks development. On a personal level it made me think of why LGBT issues are important not only in service provision but in society as a whole. I also became aware of the need to consider the safety of the people involved both for workers and also when engaging with communities and individuals.

On an organisational level I look at issues involved with partnership working, the importance of planning for sustainability and not getting caught up in the short term plans and losing sight of the future. I feel that an element of self analysis is also required as I learned something about my own knowledge and experience throughout my involvement with the LGBTEN. I look into what I know about LGBT issues and what I do not know, as well as what I had to offer the network.

West Dunbartonshire's Community Plan highlights a commitment to equality and diversity from Community Planning partners. A decision was taken by the West Dunbartonshire Community Planning Equalities Group to make raising awareness of Lesbian, Gay, Bisexual and Transgender issues a priority.

The LGBT Equality Network was established in October 2007 in response to the Community Planning Partnership Equalities Working Group's decision to look for interested parties to develop LGBT issues in West Dunbartonshire. Membership of the Network includes local and national voluntary and statutory organisations.

I became involved after the group had been established and were on their way to organising events. My line manager had been identified as a potential partner but it was agreed that it would be more appropriate for me to attend as West Dunbartonshire Council's Equality and Diversity Training Officer as I had skills and knowledge in the field of equality and diversity and training delivery. New partners are continually identified and anyone who has an interest in the LGBTEN has been invited to join or attend meetings. West Dunbartonshire Council's homeless service staff joined as statistics show that being an LGBT person can be a contributing factor to the reasons why some people become homeless. Other partners included Strathclyde Police, Unison, Streetlinks, WDC Youth Services, WDC Policy Unit and WD Violence against Women Partnership.

The majority of meetings were originally held in West Dunbartonshire Community Planning Partnership resource base in Clydebank with support from Community Support Team staff. Within two weeks of its first meeting network members had agreed a role and remit along with a programme of work including short and long term aims. A successful bid was made for funding to The Community

Regeneration Fund to fund capacity building locally around LGBT issues.

The group met initially on a monthly basis with regular contact between meetings as deadlines for programmed activities were fairly close. No actual lead role or responsibility was identified within the group and the meetings were held using a co-operative working model where those attending meetings worked by agreeing roles and task allocations depending on who was present at meetings. I believe that this informal approach initially contributed to the success and effectiveness of the groups' relationships and achievements as members were able to select roles and responsibilities that tied in with their organisations commitment to the partnership in terms of resources available and their own priorities and objectives. The group has since identified that assigning tasks to specific people with agreement will ensure that there is a balance of commitment and responsibility in future. As with all groups there can be a tendency for some people to take on more than others so this new arrangement should ensure a fairer share of tasks and involvement.

Although there were no formally elected leaders within the group some individuals were able to take on lead roles based on their knowledge, access to networks and their ability to motivate others who were perhaps less confident on LGBT issues. I believe that contributed to the success and speed of the groups' ability to achieve goals in the short term. There was an unspoken leadership within the group where individuals identified as natural leaders because of their passion and commitment to the cause as well as their knowledge and access to resources. Decisions were made democratically but there was no system for having a deciding vote should the group not be able to agree. This circumstance did not arise but that would be worth considering in future and would perhaps justify nominating a formal chairperson or lead role within the group.

Some of the network's short and long term aims were initially met through organised events which were undertaken within less than six months of being established and were partly funded by History Month Scotland. These were:

LGBT Visibility Campaign – Held in February to coincide with the LGBT History Month national campaign to raise awareness of LGBT issues and challenge homophobic attitudes. This involved producing posters and postcards that were widely distributed locally. Also two bus shelter adverts were placed in prominent areas to reach as many people as possible. Local structures such as the Titan Crane and West Dunbartonshire Council buildings also displayed rainbow flags and colours which are symbolic of the LGBT history month. This received recognition at a Parliament Reception and also a Communities Minister reception in Edinburgh Castle. I noticed some impact of the Visibility Campaign during some of the training sessions that I delivered to West Dunbartonshire Council staff as they were aware of the rainbow flag and its symbolism after the event as it was advertised widely within the organisation and in local media.

Celebrating Diversity Event for young people – The aim was to raise awareness of equality anddDiversity issues including human rights and participation. This event was organised to take place in one of the current discos that are hosted by Club T in Clydebank with a theme of celebrating equality and diversity. This was attended by 210 young people aged between 12 and 18 years old. Information stalls were available and campaign leaflets for the 'All Different All Equal' Young Scot campaign were given out. Around 50 young people expressed an interest in joining a consultation group called FUSION to involve young people in further discussion about equality and diversity issues.

Celebrating Diversity Event for all ages – This was a celebration event of equality and diversity. It was well attended by local people and workers as well as elected members. The LGBTEN members had decided to invite people from all walks of life as there was a recognition that narrowing the event to LGBT people only would perhaps not be very effective as people may not feel able to attend for a number of reasons. Perhaps safety issues, stigma and coming out to neighbours or workers would have deterred people from joining in. We felt that having an equality and diversity event with a theme of LGBT issues would be a more welcoming and safe environment for everyone. One of the main messages from the visibility campaign was that LGBT people are parents, brothers, sisters, grandparents, aunts and uncles so the openness of the event reinforced that message.

The evening consisted of speakers and a quiz with music and food. There were a number of guest speakers which included West Dunbartonshire's Provost who talked about West Dunbartonshire Councils' commitment to equality and diversity. MSP Patrick Harvie gave an overview of the Hate Crimes Bill which is progressing through Parliament since he lodged a proposal for a member's bill to recommend the introduction of a statutory aggravation law for crimes motivated by malice or ill-will on grounds of sexual orientation, transgender identity and disability in Scotland. This bill has now been introduced in the Parliament as the Offences (Aggravation by Prejudice) (Scotland) Bill in May 2008.

People's comments throughout the event were recorded on DVD to be used in further awareness raising campaigns and also as an evaluation of the LGBTEN work so far.

LGBT Awareness and Anti-Homophobia Training for Trainers – The aim of the training was to deliver LGBT awareness training and build the capacity of service providers and community members to support the local LGBT community and workforce. This was delivered to LGBTEN members by LGBT Youth Scotland Trainers. A working sub group of the LGBTEN was established to progress the training programme. By November 2008 39 members of staff from various agencies within West Dunbartonshire had received LGBT awareness training. The sub group meet on a regular basis to review training and share good practice as well as support each other.

The timing of the events that were organised tied in with national events and this enabled the partnership to network with national organisations like LGBT Youth Scotland and LGBT History Month Scotland. The momentum and pace of the group reflected the enthusiasm of the partners involved in the planning and organising of the newly established LGBTEN. Motivation for being involved in the network varied. Some members had objectives to meet as part of their roles and responsibilities in their jobs. Others had personal or emotional commitments to the aims and objectives of the network. This mix worked well as everyone had personal or professional reasons for their involvement, or both. The range of skills, knowledge and experience varied within the group and I felt that the atmosphere was a supportive one where people were able to say if they felt they needed support in any area.

During the time I was a member of the LGBTEN I was reminded of Focault's argument that "*power and knowledge are inter-related*" and that "*discourse is related to power as it operates by rules of exclusion*" (http://en.wikipedia.org/wiki/Discourse 31/12/08). Realising this enabled me to keep in mind that the language used when talking about LGBT issues could help to shape the views that people formed in society. This was important to consider when promoting the LGBTEN and particularly when designing the visibility campaign.

The Scottish Governments Attitudes to Discrimination in Scotland 2006 (Bromley and Curtice, 2006) social attitudes survey shows that trends in discriminatory attitudes towards gay men and women have decreased but have not disappeared. It was essential to remember this and consider both the emotional and physical safety of workers and the community when engaging in any activity. It was agreed that awareness raising training would always be delivered by two members of the group at any one time. This would enable trainers to support each other if they felt it necessary particularly when facing difficult or challenging attitudes or behaviour.

The training for trainers was one of the LGBTEN's short term goals to create a pool of staff to deliver awareness raising and anti-homophobia training to people throughout West Dunbartonshire. Thompson states that ".. *emancipating forms of practice need to be based on a degree of sensitivity, a raised level of awareness of how easy it can be to reinforce patterns of marginalisation unwittingly, by simply making 'common sense' assumptions.*"(1988: 82) I felt that the training had the potential to enable participants develop a critical awareness of how LGBT people become marginalised in society and to equip them with skills and knowledge to challenge both their own and other peoples 'commons sense assumptions' which lead to direct or indirect discrimination.

The timescales for planning and delivery of events and activities were quite tight from the day the network was established. The danger here was that longer term planning, particularly for the sustainability of the network, was perhaps not given enough consideration as all the member's time was focussed on meeting tight deadlines. However, some of the longer term aims were also met in the short term. The long term aim was to engage local people to be partners and be more representative of the community. It is believed that LGBT people who live in West Dunbartonshire travel to Glasgow for socialising or to gain access to specific service for LGBT people like health or advice. This may be for privacy or safety reasons but could also be because these services do not exist currently in West Dunbartonshire or are not widely advertised if they did exist. Without hard evidence of who the population are we could only assume that the numbers of LGBT people living in the area were reflective of the national UK figures.

Although it was never formalised who was taking the lead role in the network, I always assumed it was West Dunbartonshire Community Planning Partnership as they provided most of the resources in terms of access to resource bases, support workers and administration support. When the support worker from the WDCPP left mid 2008 and the resource base closed the LGBTEN membership then had to consider how it would replace the lost resources. Storage space for materials, meeting rooms and administrative support had to be found at short notice. I was able to provide storage space for the materials for the visibility campaign and the training. Fortunately the commitment of the members has enabled the network to continue however, it had quite an impact on the networks ability to function for a period of time. Perhaps in partnership working it would be appropriate to nominate a lead organisation who can offer the resources required to enable the partnership to make long term plans that ensure the sustainability and allows for the possibility that what starts as a small project can quite rapidly become a major piece of work with additional responsibilities. The LGBTEN have made identifying a lead person or agency one of its aims for 2008.

This LGBTEN multi agency work has been deemed by those involved to be very successful and is also thought to be a first in West Dunbartonshire. The LGBTEN is part of an overall bureaucratic structure in terms of the hierarchy of the Community Planning Partnership. However, it operates on a more informal basis. Huczynski and Buchanan (2001: 495) say that *"...in the twenty-first century the bureaucratic organisation will be incapable of responding sufficiently quickly to change and will not be using the innovative resources of its members"*. I feel that, given how quickly the LGBTEN was formed and was delivering on its short term objectives, the innovative resources of its members were the driving force behind the motivation to create positive change for LBGT people in West Dunbartonshire.

In terms of my own practice the learning lesson for me was that I should always be aware of how my actions can impact on LGBT people and how detrimental my actions could be if I do not consider LGBT issues when delivering services in the community. Equality legislation in terms of public service delivery has only evolved to currently place duties on local authorities to ensure they do not discriminate against people due to disability, gender and race. This should change when the proposed single Equality Bill becomes law as it will ensure that service provision is extended to sexual orientation, religion and belief and age. Meanwhile it makes sense to be pro-active to ensure that all equality strands are critically considered when delivering mainstream services.

The LGBTEN to date has not had the opportunity to fully evaluate the impact of its work so far but I managed to get testimonial evidence from people who live and or work in the area who are lesbian, gay, bisexual or transgender. They say that the impact of the visibility campaign was that their children saw the posters on the bus shelters and it helped them to understand that this was something public and local in support of LGBT people and not just something that was discussed in the home. It made them feel uplifted and felt that it would help their children as their friends would also see the public displays of support. It was also felt that the visibility of LGBT issues and support would have a positive effect on pupils who had taken parting sexual bullying classes and had discussed homophobic language and attitudes. One person said that the campaign gave them more confidence to be open about their sexuality in the community.

At present I am unable to find or produce any local statistics to show who I work with because current equal opportunities monitoring systems do not include any questions on sexual orientation. The Glasgow Community Learning Partnership has produced guidance on equal opportunities monitoring which promotes focussing monitoring on the six main equalities strands promoted by the Scottish Executive (age, disability, Ethnic origin, gender, faith and sexual orientation). They highlight Community Learning and Developments commitment to targeting activities towards the most excluded and vulnerable groups. The Scottish Government has produced guidance entitled Same

Difference as a resource for practitioners to ensure their practice is inclusive of equalities groups.

The LGBTEN worked on the assumption that there will be LGBT people within the population of West Dunbartonshire but had no hard evidence to support those assumptions. The census 2011 should include a question about sexual orientation and may provide some statistical evidence but public authorities and service providers should be identifying who they provide services to and ensuring that groups of people or communities, who have historically been excluded, marginalised or made invisible, are included. Thompson talks about the process of invisibilisation and states that "*By invisibilising relatively powerless people, dominant social groups are able to maintain their hegemony relatively unchallenged*" (1998: 83). Heterosexism is the oppressive system that excludes the needs and does not recognise the cultures of anyone who is not heterosexual and therefore maintains the notion that people are or should be heterosexual. With that comes a set of invisible or hidden privileges. Without those privileges the needs and identities of LGBT people remain neglected and hidden resulting in inequity of opportunity in public and private sectors of their lives.

In 2006 the LGBT Hearts and Minds Agenda Group was set up to look at the impact of negative attitudes today on LGBT people and to come up with recommendations to address this. It has been acknowledged that equality law has progressed over the past 30 years but that negative attitudes still exist that can prevent LGBT people from participating fully in society and achieving their potential. The Hearts and Minds Agenda Group produced a report that was published by the Scottish Government Equality Unit and recommended ways to address changing attitudes. This report was called "*Challenging Prejudice: Changing Attitudes Towards Lesbians, Gay, Bisexual and Transgender People in Scotland*" and was presented to the Scottish Government in February 2008. Recommendations from the report will be built into local authority single outcome agreements which tie in with national outcomes and indicators as well as being considered at a strategic level by the Scottish Government. This should ensure that LGBT equality becomes mainstreamed and part of every agenda in public services.

The future of equality and fairness for LGBT people has been changing since the creation of the Equality and Human Rights Commission in 2007. The ECHR now have the power to enforce anti discriminatory legislation relating to LGBT people and to ensure that public service providers comply with these laws. This is the first time that there has been a Commission that covers sexual orientation. The proposed new single Equality Bill will also bring changes in terms of service provision as it will include duties for public service providers to ensure that they actively promote equality for LGBT people. The LGBTEN will play an important role in West Dunbartonshire in ensuring that LGBT people get included in the processes of change within the local authority area and are kept visible on the agendas of key partners and stakeholders.

The outcomes identified by the LGBTEN for the future are to *"create a safe and inclusive environment for LGBT people living and working in West Dunbartonshire and ensuring better outcomes for young people living in West Dunbartonshire."* Given the climate of change the LGBTEN is a long awaited resource that has the potential to make a difference to the lives of West Dunbartonshire's LGBT people.

Commentary

This study highlights work on LGBT issues that is often ignored by mainstream community organisations. It demonstrates how systems, processes and resources can be creatively and effectively utilised if local workers are committed enough to make it happen.

It might be suggested that the work was successful in developing a range of activities in a short period of time because of the flexible and informal structure that was adopted. Also mentioned is the importance of personal reflection on practice.

Practice Study 3

HOPE: support to offenders, prisoners and their families

Janice Quinn

Abstract

This study is based on a group of parents and their children. It promoted the parents as a self help group focused on developing play activities for their children. The work is discussed from a variety of practice perspectives.

The Study

HOPE, based in the East End of Glasgow is an organisation which offers a variety of support to offenders, prisoners and their families. Over the past seven years I have worked throughout Glasgow and Dunbartonshire in various capacities within HOPE and have many years experience working with those leaving prison and with families of those serving the sentence in the community. For the past three and half years I have managed a project which delivers support to families affected by addictions and imprisonment. The project also supports prisoners as they return to their families and communities. I have witnessed firsthand the difficulties parents and children are faced with everyday as they try to survive in communities affected by poverty and other ills, and surrounded by others in the same predicament. In this study I will attempt to describe, reflect on and evaluate my practice against the background of good community values practice and current developments, and demands.

The main aim of the work was to encourage parents to engage with their children through play. This idea was born from my experience in working with families and observing the lack of positive play interaction within families. This work was used as a learning experience for the organisation as it prepared to deliver a new project focussing on Parenting and Relationships.

A steering group of six was formed by gathering parents from HOPE and other local organisations in the East End of Glasgow. The remit of the steering group was three fold, firstly to encourage the parents to organise an event around the area of play, secondly to provide opportunities to take part in play activities and finally to look at barriers that prevent parents from engaging with their children through play. The long term aims of the work undertaken were to build relationships within families, to help build sustainable communities and to encourage inclusion. It was hoped that participants in the steering group would take ownership of the group and begin to influence the services provided in their area.

The approach I used for the placement was rooted in the theory and methods of Paulo Freire. His own life experiences working in community settings with the poor, and later as an educator, led him to the theory developed and described in his book Pedagogy of the Oppressed (Freire 1996). Participants and teacher become partners in exploring together why things happen, and questioning their own situations and that of the wider world. Traditional ways of education where the teacher imparts knowledge which is stored and retained in a banking process give way to a collaborative sharing of knowledge and skills between the group leader or facilitator and the group.

Central to Freire's approach was its problem-posing method. A common problem within a community is explored and by constantly questioning and exploring it, solutions can be found. It is not the teacher telling the learner the answer, but rather the teacher and learner sharing knowledge and using it to bring about change for their local community. It is rooted in the concrete experiences of people and by inviting participants to reflect critically on their life and circumstances, to learn from their collective experiences. A new consciousness is created and their new knowledge and understanding is liberating. Reaching awareness called conscientisation is described by Wright Mills (1959 cited by Ledwith 2005) as being when "*problems move from being private troubles to public issues*". By challenging attitudes and social structures that maintain the status quo it moves from being action based learning, and becomes deeply political as it demands collective action for change to overthrow systems that allow the continuing enslaving of the oppressed. The pillars of Popular Education are empowerment, collective action, social justice and transformative change. They were also the intended outcomes of our modest venture.

It was important to bring together the values and practice principles of The National Occupational Standards for Community Development Work. One of the Practice Principles, Self-determination, states "*Valuing the concerns or issues that communities identify as their starting points*". Another Practice Principle under the heading of Sustainable Communities is "*promoting the empowerment of individuals and communities*". (PAULO, 2003: 2) I found these to be particularly relevant to my own values and attitudes as I planned an initiative that had at its core the important part played by 'working and learning together' in community development. I tried to share with the steering group an understanding of the meaning and importance of this from the very beginning.

The National Occupational Standards highlight the place of dialogue in bringing about change, and that the best path to achieving it is by listening to the stories and concerns that people have and building trust. A good example of how to do this is found in Freire's approach where reality is discovered in a dialogue that pays attention to the collection of individual experiences. As these are shared, patterns are identified as community concerns, critical knowledge is increased, collective responsibility is acknowledged, and planning for action can happen. During this project I tried to adopt Freire's approach and participated in a lot of dialogue with the parents not only in the steering group but also the parents who attended the events that took place during the placement.

The National Occupational Standards indicates the role of reflection throughout the process of community development. For Freire, reflection and action are valid and effective when they go together. Planning and action followed by reviewing is a continuous cycle. An important principle of Community Development is that the community worker be a reflective practitioner "*promoting and supporting individual and collective learning through reflection on practice*". (PAULO, 2003: 2) During my placement, I initially forgot to engage the group in reflection, however, as the work proceeded, I did engage the group and saw how effective and empowering reflection is.

By reflecting on my work practice I feel that I have developed my practice by trying to monitor and evaluate my progress and the progress of the group against the values and practice principles of community work. Respect is an important value for me. I always treated the group with respect and encouraged them to do the same with each other. In the group, we started talking about what ground rules were needed and the group identified respect for each other as a requirement. Others were to respect individual opinion, to maintain confidentiality, to ensure that only one person spoke at a time and always to have mobile phones on silent. Racism and sectarianism were added in the second week after one member made reference to 'pakkies', 'chinkies' and 'huns'. These rules were policed by the group itself. As group leader, I am aware that one of my roles is to ensure that the group rules were used effectively. By revisiting the rules in week two I reinforced for the group a way of dealing with challenging behaviour.

Participation by the group started in the first meeting through discussion where everyone was encouraged to contribute and share their opinions. Roles and responsibilities were agreed, as tasks were identified and shared out, some for individuals and others for small units working together. The group gathered the information required and fed their research back to the group. Decisions were based on group preferences, taking into account the needs of people who would be taking part but who were not part of the steering group. Group development was only possible because I went to each session with a plan. I became more aware as the work progressed that if I was not well prepared the group could drift away from the task and spend the meeting chatting. My learning from this experience is that participation in a group has to be planned and cannot just happen.

I had discussed with my manager that some funding would be helpful for group expenses, to enable them to carry out and make a success of the plan. I submitted a costing and a budget of four hundred pounds was agreed to cover the activity that the group would organise. In the event, after researching a number of activities, deliberating the positives, negatives and appropriateness of each activity, the group decided on a visit to Glasgow Science Centre.

Other activities agreed and organised were working with Theatre Nemo and participating in Community Football. Theatre Nemo is a charity set up to give a voice to social issues, especially mental health. They had asked HOPE to work in partnership with them to deliver ten weekly creative workshops in the East End of Glasgow. The workshops would encourage parents and children to meet together weekly on Saturday afternoons and provided the opportunity to take part in storytelling, learn how to make music using a computer, and make an animated DVD.

This last task involved starting with a wire frame, using different colours of plasticine to create a figure, add a face, hair and other features. The final stage is to make an animated DVD using the figures created by all the children. The concept at the heart of the workshops is to have fun, build confidence and develop communication skills. Community Football coaching course was the final activity. Nine Children participated in a course over five days during the Easter school break run by both Celtic and Rangers football clubs. The children loved all three activities. The parents were delighted with all three. One father commented "*he is like a different wee boy, since he took part in the football. He is a lot more confident about making friends and mixing with other children*".

Fairness and equality are principles of community development that are very real for the group I worked with. They are often treated without fairness and this is something I feel really strongly about. Their feelings and needs are sometimes not taken seriously, and they are often talked down to. They have a well developed sense of justice for themselves and others but lack power and knowledge to challenge.

Power has more than one face. I think of it as having freedom, skills, and knowledge to decide and accomplish an end. Power "over" to me has an undertone of domination and class. I like the distinction by Mills (cited by Butcher 2007: 23) about "*the power of non decision-making which the powerful can use to ensure that potentially difficult issues do not get onto decision-making agendas in the first place*".

The empowerment of the disadvantaged is the primary concern of community development. I tried to empower the group by stressing that every person has rights. However, I am aware that I was not always empowering. Theatre Nemo asked HOPE to work in partnership with them and we agreed roles and responsibilities. Three weeks into the ten week course the venue was changed without consultation with HOPE. The biggest casualty of this was a single parent who brought his four boys to the group. Two of them have a disability and are hyperactive. Because the premises were smaller, Theatre Nemo felt it could not accommodate three of the children, and excluded the two boys and also the youngest who was three, despite the fact that I had discussed the family situation with its staff as part of our agreement prior to the start of the intervention. I expressed my disappointment to

Theatre Nemo, and intimated that the group was upset by the treatment of the family.

After reflection and consultation with my supervisor, I realise that this event should have been dealt with by the group.had taken action unilaterally instead of sharing the decision and course of action with the group, and to that extent missed an opportunity to empower them. We discussed this together, and although it is something they found difficult to "*get their head around*", my mistake gave them a different slant on what community development practice is.

My role changed working with this group. I went from someone who supported and advocated for them to one who was guiding them to take responsibility for working with each other to achieve a definite aim. I found this difficult at first because I felt quite protective of them. I was reluctant to put too much on to them but as the weeks went by this changed when I realised that they were not only capable of accepting responsibility but thrived on it. I tried to get them to realise that they had some skills and to match their skills to the tasks. I encouraged them in everything they did and tried to reinforce their growing confidence by praising them and acknowledging their progress each week. I realise my role is important and at times I am not sure I managed to make clear to the group the reasons why it is good practice to do things in a certain way. An example of this is that I failed to explain initially the reasons for monitoring and evaluation and its value, although we were doing it every week.

Despite this, the group learned a lot of skills during the project. Research skills were gained by using the telephone, internet and by visiting venues to assess them. The group accessed local resources in the library, finding out information on groups and organisations. Every one of them decided to join the library. As a group they worked collectively to achieve their aim.

All of the interventions that took place during my placement were successful to some extent. Overall I think the group learned that they had existing skills that could be transferred into something that in fact was good community practice because they were following a method/plan that helped them achieve what they set out to do. At the beginning of my placement, the group members were inconsistent in turning up on time, although we had agreed a time. I revisited the earlier agreement and the time was changed. I was pleased that the group worked collectively. The outing and other activities they organised were great successes and they could see this was a benefit to them as a group and to their children. I found that my group work skills have been improved during this placement as I challenged the group members to be responsible in the group. By challenging the group, I realise that I was encouraging active participation. Tett comments that:

> "*The active participation of ordinary people in creating the projects that shape themselves, as well as the communities in which they live, provides a reason for working together with others to secure trusting relations within the community. The possibility of shared understanding requires not only the valuing of others but also the creation of communities in which mutuality and thus the conditions for learning can flourish*" (2006: 67).

I realise that this does not happen without challenge and this has been something that I have learned during this work.

Regular meetings with my supervisor helped me reflect on my practice. Through discussion I was able to come to a realisation of my strengths and weaknesses. I took on board her constructive criticism and tried to adapt my practice where needed. Encouraged by her recognition of the good points in my practice, I was able to have a group discussion reflecting on the success of the group. This helped me appreciate the value of supervision not only for me, but also for the groups that I work with. Completing reflective accounts also helped me to monitor and evaluate my practice.

> "*Self criticism is an act of frankness, courage, comradeship and awareness of our responsibilities, a proof of our will to accomplish and to accomplish properly... To criticise oneself is to reconstruct oneself within oneself in order to serve better*" (Amilcar Cabral cited by Hope & Timmel 1995, Book 2: 81).

I absolutely agree with this statement but found the process difficult, challenging and really emotional. I considered myself a reflective practitioner but it was evident that I need to reflect a lot more. I am now more aware that engaging in reflection is an integral part of community development work and I intend to continue keeping reflective accounts of my practice.

I tried to follow the LEAP (Learning Evaluation and Planning) produced for the Scottish Government (2007) as a framework for monitoring and evaluation. It is recognised as a process that is used widely, is adaptable to different circumstances, and is seen as a model of good practice in community development. I found it helpful as it reassured me about the validity and reliability of the approach and interventions I was using. It is a cyclical process of five steps which when followed properly is a good guide for achieving and monitoring outcomes by tracking and measuring the difference you are making. Its five steps are agreeing outcomes, identifying indicators, action planning, monitoring and evaluation.

An example of a lapse in its use on my part is the Theatre Nemo incident mentioned above, which led me to engage in a situation that appeared to present a contradiction between my values and my practice. I wanted the boys to be treated fairly. I was clear that to improve the interaction between parent and child Theatre Nemo would be a resource. I intended to use this resource for the four children in this family. I was clear that the methods I would use would be engaging parent and children in play. However, when the children became unruly and disruptive, I became their childminder. It was only when I shared my diary entry with my manager that I realised I had contradicted my practice values. I am aware that there are potential contradictions that I sometimes engage in. I would offer a lift to a group member in my car if the weather was very bad. I am now becoming aware that this is bad practice. Such behaviour leaves me open to challenge and I have to start thinking more deeply about my actions and the consequences for the organisation that employs me.

Had I made more reference to the LEAP model when dealing with the children, I would not have engaged in the behaviour described. The model refers at the beginning to what the need is. Even by answering that question, I would have behaved differently. The outcome I wanted was to allow father and son to get time together without the other three children. I lost sight of how I would know that the intervention had made a difference to the family. I did not establish reliable indicators, nor assess outcomes other than what I hoped for. I did not think through and plan sufficiently. Proper use and interrogation of the five step cycle would have helped keep me focussed. I can also refer to the values and principles of community development for guidance. It is interesting to note that the roles I adopt state I am working 'with' people. If I remembered this, there would be fewer contradictions in my practice as I sometimes work '*for*' people rather than '*with*' them.

A more appropriate action for the family mentioned above would have been to work with a partner organisation. I could have supported the father in finding childcare for his three younger children. This would have allowed him to spend quality time with his oldest son in a relaxed manner. He could have improved his interaction with his son and he would have let his son engage in play and act like the 10 year old that he is. Instead of this, the father was anxious about his other three sons and his 10 year old once again did not get his father's full attention. Interestingly, I had spoken to this father about respite care, but I did not think about it before or during this activity. Theatre Nemo, in its risk assessment, had recognised a fundamental fact that I had not. I lost sight of the overall aim of the intervention, which was to allow the Father and the eldest son to spend time together. I had not taken into account the wisdom of allowing the other children to continue at a risk to themselves, and to the detriment of the others in the group.

There appears to be an almost infinite potential for contradictions with community development work because of the tensions that can exist within communities and between different organisations. This can arise because of differing values, approaches, cultures, politics, priorities, power relationships and issues where feelings and expectations vary. Within organisations themselves all these circumstances can exist and the pressure that differences create can be detrimental to the work, to the organisation, or to the worker. Similarly these clashes can arise with client groups where the opinions, behaviours, attitudes, and sometimes lack of structure in their lives can make it difficult to plan and achieve quality outcomes.

Some of these dangers can be avoided by the individual worker or the organisation by a clear statement and practice of community values and principles, by keeping close to good practice as defined by the National Occupational Standards, by transparency, and by following a reliable process of planning action and review through reflection. Training has an important part to play in achieving these outcomes, as has supervision and regulation. Most important of all is consistency and striving to create trust and respect in every circumstance.

I discovered that one single model does not fulfil the needs of communities. I think however, that this is not a criticism but strength of community practice. A worker should be able to adopt and adapt models as required to meet the needs of the community that you are working with.

The popular education model of Paulo Freire sees the oppressed coming to accept as normal the boundaries that they impose on themselves, and the way forward for Freire was through education which can liberate. This was my starting point with my group. Their experience was as an oppressed group, in many ways excluded from mainstream society. I am fully committed to this model as that which defines best what I think, and feel, and how I act in my approach and practice as far as education and learning is concerned. A vital part of my work is empowering and helping disadvantaged individuals and groups to cast off the shackles and liberate themselves from unfair boundaries, self imposed or imposed by the structures and circumstances they have inherited. In Freire's model, the teacher is the community worker, the animator, who poses questions inviting the group/individual to reflect on situations in the light of their own experiences. By encouraging the learner to discover the personal and political reality, this education is liberating and transformatory. Beyond the attachment I feel towards it as a learning and liberating agent, I see value in other models for complementing and adding further dimensions in meeting needs and achieving outcomes.

All through my placement I have been very aware of the need for improvements in people's quality of life that is sustainable. I have tried to ensure that the work was seen as a pioneer for HOPE as well as a requirement for me, and have tried to approach, monitor, and record it in a way that it could be seen as making a real difference to the participants.

I was surprised that I enjoyed it so much and that those who took part were so enthusiastic, and eager for more. It was with this in mind that I suggested to them that we celebrate success by a gathering of all who had taken part, our partner organisations, and the managers and staff of HOPE. The group took responsibility for setting up a display of the photographs of all the play activities, catering for the buffet, and acting as guides and promoters of the need for this and similar ventures to be continued. I am now convinced that sustainability should be second only to empowerment in importance in achieving lasting change through community development.

> *"The dominant ideology of the powerful in society gives rise to discrimination that becomes structurally imbedded in its institutions. Any change that aims to be transformative, rather than tokenistic or ameliorative, has to target the root causes of injustice not just the systems, and this involves structural change"* (Ledwith 2005: 94).

The National Occupational Standards give clear guidance on the role and the expected practice of a community development worker. The standards are the guidebook for my practice, and it is only by engaging in practice that the standards become real. It will take me a longer time than this placement to be able to feel that I am using the standards well or appropriately at all times.

Of the developments mentioned above, I would continue to use all of them in my future practice. There are particular aspects of each that I find useful. Paulo Freire's work starts with people and where they are. It allows people to bring their own experience to a group. The group members all have skills and Freire's model reminds me to keep this at the forefront of my mind when working with a group. Without this thought, I might rule the group rather than facilitate the group.

As I finish my involvement with the group I am aware that the following training needs still exist. They include learning more about the theory and methods of community engagement, involving service users, building networks and partnership working, and sharing good practice. I am aware of the need to include monitoring and reviewing at the beginning, middle and end of a project. My skills of working with groups will improve through practice and I have to trust and respect their skills and experience, instead of trying to protect them. All of these would not only help me avoid contradictions, but deliver the outcomes the clients and the organisation needs and deserves.

Commentary

Underpinning this work is a strong commitment to the values of community development. It is clearly located in a range of overlapping frameworks; where private concerns are linked to public issues, a wider popular education / transformation approach, and also within the National Occupational Standards. The writer argues for flexibility in approaches and demonstrates the importance of being able to think about the work from different perspectives.

This is clearly aspirational work that recognises that although major changes may be desired, the reality for much of practice is small scale and local. Nevertheless significant sustainable changes for small groups and individuals can be achieved.

The worker also demonstrates the importance of self reflection, systematic evaluation of practice and continually learning lessons from practice.

Practice Study 4

Local Authority supported youth work

Steven Gilfoyle

Abstract

This practice study is located with a youth group receiving conventional local authority youth work practice. The author raises a number of critical questions on the assumptions underpinning this practice.

The Study

This practice study reports on work within Culture and Sport Glasgow's (CSG) Youth Services department's South West Area Team. CSG South West team are based in the Rowan Park hub in Drumoyne and work throughout the south west of Glasgow. CSG are a city wide organization who as a wing of Glasgow City Council are responsible for delivering services in the following areas: Arts and Museums, Libraries and Community Facilities, Sporting occasions and events, and social renewal initiatives and events and according to CSG literature includes:

Community services and play
Service Development (Sport)
Community Learning (Adult)
Education and Access (Museums, learning centres)
Youth Services (young people aged 12 -18)
Client management role for capital projects
Event planning and policy
Strategic infrastructure planning
Main link with city's physical and economic regeneration strategies

The study looks at my role and my work with a group of young people from the local community in Drumoyne, a social excluded area in the south side of Glasgow. In particular my work supporting the group to form a service users committee, support the group to identify aims and objectives, and launch a new user lead the club initiative called 'Beat Street'; a youth club with music and dance as some of the main activities, as the young people themselves identified these activities as something they would want to participate in.

This study evaluates and challenges the potential contradictions in values and practice, by giving an example of a situation where the values and principles of community development were not practical when applied in this specific youth work situation and/or at this stage in a community with this type of demographic makeup. It will critically review and use current developments in community work practice, giving an example of different approaches, which methods I had chosen for my work and why.

On a personal level I value freedom, equality, justice, the right to have a say, the right to an opinion, equality of opportunity regardless of background, the right to participate in society, the right to work, the right to contribute. These personal values of mine align well with the values and principles from the National Occupational Standards in Community Development Work (PAULO 2003). From my 8 years of experience of working within communities and groups I don't find that working with groups has changed my values in any way, and have only underlined, clarified and strengthened my own personal beliefs. This is one reason why I find so much personal satisfaction when working within the community.

To help my practice be more effective and remain focused and on track I normally employ the LEAP framework (Scottish Government, 2007) as my method of monitoring and evaluation as this is the method I am most experienced in using. LEAR is also the evaluation method favoured by our current funders (Community Planning Partnership).

LEAP works by giving the group / community questions to consider, such as:

- What things need to change? – What aims and objectives have the group identified collectively
- How will we know it has changed? – How will we measure the outcomes the group aims to achieve?
- How will we change it? – What methods and strategy will the

group employ to reach its objective?
- How will we monitor what we do? – What system will the group use to monitor and evaluate its effectiveness?
- How will we learn from our experience? - What systems for review, strengths and weaknesses of the strategy, what can be improved.

The LEAP framework works in a cycle. It is an ongoing process that will monitor the implementation of our plans and allow us to learn what does and what doesn't work. Once these questions are answered by the group, they can use this information to devise a strategy or framework against which an activity or action is planned, monitored and its progress evaluated.

CSG employs a similar method for the evaluation of the effectiveness of work within the community and when working with / supporting groups. This is called How Good Is Our Community Learning and Development (HGIOCLD). Once I was familiar with HGIOCLD I recognized that it had a very similar methodology, values and principles to other methods of community development and community capacity building, with key themes such as:

- Work with communities to identify their needs
- Developing skills and confidence
- Promoting participation in community affairs
- Assisting communities to exercise power and influence
- Monitoring and evaluation as part of building community capacity
- Community achievement

In addition, all procedures had to comply with CSG's other policies including health and safety, equality and diversity, working with volunteers, child protection and data protection.

As a worker with a popular education approach to my methods I firmly believe that the learning process is a two way thing, and as such I try to keep an open mind when working with new groups, and I try to avoid if possible a traditional teacher / student power relationship / situation because of the narrative nature of the traditional delivery method for imparting and sharing of knowledge. Paulo Freire defined this method of delivery of knowledge as the '*Banking Method*' of education, or as he saw it, another method for the control and the manipulation of the masses by the oppressors.

The banking method of education is the basis of the traditional teacher / student roles, and it leaves no or little room for the development of the creative consciousness of the students, thus maintaining the power deficit between the oppressed and the oppressor;

> "*..The banking concept of education regarding men as adaptable, manageable beings. The more students work at storing the deposits entrusted to them, the less they develop the critical consciousness which would result from their intervention in the world as transformers of that world*" (Friere 1993).

On one of the first times that the group had gathered collectively was for an introductory session with the group to identify and set their own aims and objectives. As young people have their own culture and identity they may have different views and ideas from us adults, and I wanted to make sure that they had an opportunity to express themselves comfortably, but due to the young ages of the group, the lack of confidence from some members and a lack of understanding of the process this took more guiding and support from me than I had originally prepared for or anticipated.

I quickly adapted my role and relationship with the group, and my role changed from facilitator to youth leader. The role of a youth leader is not to be impartial but to educate offer positive advice and guidance to the young people. I think this is similar to community development principles in general, but with more of an emphasis on skills and leadership.

After reflection on my role and the initial session I had with the young people I realised that my previous experiences of working with groups had influenced the way I thought the session would pan out. I now understand after reflection and research on the matter that youth work requires a slightly different set of skills and values, and can sometimes require different methods and approaches when working with groups, because ultimately, youth work is about helping young people acquire the skills that they will need to successfully navigate modern urban life.

This aligns with current youth work policies and theories which suggest that:

> *"youth work changes lives. It provides opportunities for young people in a wide range of settings including sport, the arts and the community. It helps them develop the personal skills they need to make a success of their lives.*
>
> *It allows them to influence and shape their lives and the services available to them. And it allows them to put something back into their communities. There are few more important investments than in the future of young people, and few better ways of delivering change than through good youth work."* Charles Clarke, Secretary of State for Education and Skills, 2002 (foreword to Transforming Youth Work).

This quote demonstrates the importance of youth work in a community development context and clarified my role in the youth work process. This allowed me to be more prepared for our next group session where I gave the group examples instead of leaving the questions I asked open, and I lead the meeting more as this is the is expected of a worker in that environment with a similar group.

During the next sessions I took a slightly more authoritarian approach with the group than I had at first hoped or anticipated. Although in retrospect it makes sense that a group of young people from very different backgrounds and from a socially excluded area will need extra support and guidance, during what has been defined by Tuckman (in Hannigan 2005: 28) as the '*forming stage*'. Tuckman argues that a group at the beginning of the cycle of group dynamics are more inclined to act independently and are less team focused. As such any group at this stage will need to employ strategies to stay focused.

This next meeting was more productive and the young people said they found it more enjoyable. The young people seemed more comfortable when they were given a little more direction and support through the decision making process, and the use of examples and role play made it more interactive and untimely understandable for everyone. I conducted short thumbs up thumbs down evaluation to find out if the young people had enjoyed the session and if they had felt they had learned anything useful to which the responses were a lot more positive than in the first session.

Another part of the evaluation process was a short discussion with the staff and volunteers every night after the club had ended to find out how they had felt it had went, and to suggest and listen to others suggestions for how the service may be improved for the next night. This was a good method of monitoring and evaluation as it allowed it to happen while it was still fresh in everyone's head (some of the workers I wouldn't see again till the following week).

CSG also required their own internal monitoring and this consisted of me as leader completing a monitoring form and rating how I felt things went such as the quality of the youth work delivered, comments from service users and the use of resources.

The main focus of my work with the young people was to support them to form a service users committee, and to find out what type of activities they would like to take part in. This included what services and resources they required, and to help and support the young people to work towards achieving the aims and objectives they collectively identified.

As a community development practitioner I firmly believe that the values and standards of Community Development work, as defined in the National Occupational Standards in Community Development work (PAULO 2003) are there as tools to aid us in our work to support communities towards their aims and objectives.

These values such as:

- Democracy - where the power is shared, everyone can have a say
- Participation – where everyone has the right to participate or have their say in the decisions that may affect them,
- Self determination- where groups and communities can identify what is important to them,
- The Freirean approach of 'starting where people are at' or starting from a grass roots level,

As it was the young people themselves who identified the need for the youth club, I was aiming for the club to be a user lead initiative where the young people themselves would have a say and not just tokenistic in the aims and objectives of the group. I thought that CSG would not be keen on a user lead youth club as they seem to have more of a top down agenda when it comes to youth provision in the area, but after a discussion with my supervisors they agreed that the success or other wise of the club depended on how satisfied the users were with the service and that they would vote with their feet and not attend the club if they were not happy. Unfortunately I was also told by CSG that there was no budget for activities and resources, but staff (youth workers) would be made available on the night.

This I felt was a form of control from CSG. The objective is to form a user lead youth service were the young people identify their own aims and objectives and what types of activities they would like to take place in the club. But ultimately the young people would need to ask the people in control of budgets and the resources if their aims and objectives were acceptable to them and is money available. CSG has huge budgets and resources, but possibly felt it was too risky to support a user lead youth group in the initial stages where it needs most support.

After doing some informal research by speaking to local people, teachers and pupils in local schools, uniformed youth groups and community groups etc it was clear that young people had very rarely accessed the hall previously. Apparently this was because the young people felt that there was no activities taking place, or nothing that they wanted to take part in was happening at the hall. After speaking to several groups of young people and finding out what type of activities young people would like to take part and in some initial feedback from the group and the wider community I identified resources and volunteers from within the community who would help out the group by supplying some of the resources and services the young people originally asked for in the centre, such as DJ equipment and street dancing. As attending the club is voluntary these are activities that designed to attract young people to the club, and in this they were successful with 32 young people registered with the club on the first night.

It is important as a community development practitioner to keep up to date and informed with relevant policies, procedures and developments. In March 2008 the new updated National Occupational Standard for Youth Work were released, and the purpose of youth work as defined within in the document was:

> *"Enable young people to develop holistically, working with them to facilitate their personal, social and educational development, to allow them to develop their voice, influence and place in society and reach their full potential"* – (LLUK, 2008).

The focus on the update seems to be on the defining of the core skills, values and beliefs that are required to be an effective youth worker and there is a far greater number than in the previous version, but there is also a clear move in the update towards partnership working and strengthening links between youth work and the wider community, and require outcomes such as:

- Identify key contacts and agencies within the local community who are appropriate towards developing and promoting awareness of your organisation's youth work activities

- Develop and maintain a network of contacts within the local community, ensuring that they have an accurate idea of your knowledge, skills and experience relating to youth work, and the services that your organisation provides

- Promote the benefits of youth work, and of working in partnership with your organisation, to the mutual advantage of their and also your own objectives

- Identify and respect the aims and objectives of others in the community, recognising when their priorities may not always coincide with your own

- Create opportunities to be involved positively with the local community (LLUK, 2008).

Also included in the update is an outcome to "*Encourage young people to broaden their horizons to be active citizens*". This is a good concept in theory, as it aims to encourage young people to be more active in the community and thus encourages and supports community development, but if active citizenship means that a person exercises both their rights and responsibilities in a balanced way, there needs to be a clear indication of what those rights and responsibilities are.

A problem with trying to applying this concept is that although our rights are often written down as part of laws and policies, our responsibilities are not as clearly defined, and there may be disagreements amongst the young people as to what the responsibilities are. As adults we can have difficulty in understanding the parameters and concept of citizenship, and as such this must be even more difficult for young people to understand. Unless there is a clear definition of what a young person's rights and responsibilities are there is always going to be confusion over the issue.

For instance, trying to convince a young person from a disadvantaged background, that they have the same rights and responsibilities of a young person from a more affluent background would certainly be a challenge, and is also misleading for the young people. It can also obscure the true issues that may affect some young people.

These young people from a disadvantaged background are the victims of structural inequality by an unfair system of power, and until that is addressed it will be difficult to truly employ active citizenship as another method towards community development and individual empowerment, as untimely they have very little input into the allocation of resources.

To be an active citizen you need to be informed, you need to know how and where to participate and you may need to be trained. These issues can all be tackled, but before this can happen some fundamental problems that take place within some communities need to be addressed, such as poverty, bad housing conditions, unemployment, lack of skills, numeracy and literacy issues, a lack of local services and amenities, and on an individual level, people have a lack of confidence and a lack of self belief that they can achieve positive change in their own lives.

You can think of a community as a collective and relate it to Maslow (1943) and his hierarchy of needs theory which states that a person's basic needs are:

- Biological and Physiological needs – air, food, drink, shelter, warmth, sex, sleep, etc.

- Safety needs – protection from elements, security, order, law, limits, stability, etc.
- Belongingness and Love needs – work group, family, affection, relationships, etc.
- Esteem needs – self-esteem, achievement, mastery, independence, status, dominance, prestige, managerial responsibility, etc.
- Self-Actualization needs – realizing personal potential, self-fulfillment, seeking personal growth and peak experiences.

Until a communities basic needs are met and the major issues that affect communities are addressed we as workers are best serving the community by identifying the priority issues and working with the community by helping them identify a strategy to alleviate some of the issues that affect them and ultimately prevent them from achieving active citizenship.

I will summarise this line of thought with quote from Paulo Freire:

> "*it is absolutely essential that the oppressed participate in the revolutionary process with an increasingly critical awareness of their role as Subjects of the transformation. If they are drawn into the process as ambiguous beings, partly themselves and partly the oppressors housed within them-and if they come to power still embodying that ambiguity imposed on them by the situation of oppression-it is my contention that they will merely imagine they have reached power*" (Freire 1993).

Ultimately to encourage active citizenship is to encourage sustainable communities and community development, but this can only happen when structural inequality has been eradicated and although there is a strong link with an individual's rights and responsibilities and active citizenship to community development and sustainability, at the moment there is not enough information and support available within the community to encourage the active citizenship process to fully develop.

Until there is more clarification on what active citizenship really involves, what the responsibilities and requirements of active citizenship are, and until there are clearly defined mechanisms and systems are in place to encourage participation in the process, there is a danger we as workers can lose sight of the real issues that may affect communities, while trying to encourage active citizenship as an outcome.

I personally will tread carefully when approaching this issue in my practice, and I will always seek the latest information and guidance that is available from local, national and international agencies and networks.

Commentary

The author locates this practice within a traditional local authority agency / community planning setting. The nature of this intervention is described. However, the author raises a number of critical questions around the value base of youth work and community development work practice, and how this fits with the risk adverse and conservative approach to practice by the agency.

The author also raises questions on the assumptions (from agency, LLUK, Government, etc) that youth work takes place with uncontested social norms and ignores structural disadvantage, inequalities and oppression.

Practice Study 5

North Glasgow men's group: community allotment

John Bernklow

Abstract

This study looks at the development of a community based men's group. The group was established as part of a wider project tackling social exclusion and isolation. The developmental focus of the group was through a community gardening project.

The Study

This case study is a study in progress; it's about our journey together, where we started from, where we're at and where we hope to go. It describes the building of community capital and social inclusion through the development of an allotment in north Glasgow. It is situated firmly within current discourse around urban agriculture.

I explain how a group of men with an idea, became a shared vision. How that shared vision enabled them to transform a previously thriving allotment that had been allowed to become derelict, overgrown, a rubbish strewn piece of land, into a once again productive community asset.

I see this physical transformation of the allotment as a metaphor for the men's own transformation, that is through their discussions, observations, insights, experiences and the actions they have taken, they have come to reaffirm that they are persons of value, that they are an asset to the group and the wider community, they are men that are capable of bringing about positive change within their lives and also in the lives of others.

There are many lessons that can be gleaned from this work but I would emphasise five that I feel are particularly relevant to practice:

- We all have abilities that come out of a life lived; be open to recognising them, use them, share them and build upon them.
- Community learning and development, that is transformative practice, does not need to be compromised by the need to secure external funding – fundraising can be supported through other means. This act in itself can be empowering.
- Work may start off as exclusive 'this is our project' but sustainability soon requires the sharing of ideas, resources and collective action.
- Participative practice is a process; there is a balance between participation and directing. Developing trust and knowledge means that the balance of power will reside within the participants.
- Horticulture set within the community can be used as a vehicle for community capacity building

I work part time for Rosemount Lifelong Learning in Royston, North Glasgow as a men's development worker. Rosemount Lifelong Learning is a community managed charitable organisation providing childcare and education for women and men wishing to return to the labour market. It aims to reduce poverty by providing high quality childcare and increasing lifelong learning opportunities in an approachable and supportive community setting.

Since September 2006 I have developed and run the North Glasgow Men's Group (NGMG). This is a group that is open to all men. Its main aim is to break the cycle of male social exclusion and increase men's self esteem by developing men's wellbeing through participation in various group activities that the men themselves identify, one to one work and individual and group goal setting. The men I work with live in an area that is recognised as being in the worst 5% in Scotland in terms of income, employment, health and education deprivation. Underpinning this work is a community development model that believes that men's well being is determined by current social, economic and environmental factors. So borrowing from the Australian Unity Wellbeing Index the men and I were able to explore and come to articulate our understanding as to what wellbeing meant.

- Your health
- Your personal relationships
- How safe you feel
- Your standard of living
- What you are achieving in life
- Feeling part of the community, and
- Your future security

Australian Unity Wellbeing Index

It follows that there is an onus within the group to try and bring about change not only in their own lives but also in the factors that contribute to that wellbeing.

The group at this moment is funded through the Links Foundation the charitable arm of Working Links. Previous funders have been pulled together by North Glasgow Healthy Living Community and Equal a European Social Fund (ESF) Community Initiative.

About two thirds of the group are referred from addiction agencies, mental health practitioners/agencies, social work and equal access to employment workers. The other third are self-referrals that have come to the group through word of mouth or through marketing.

One of the strengths of the group lies in its diversity, it offers the members the opportunity of sharing their life experiences in their own language that on first thought may seem disparate but on reflection shows a commonality that comes out of isolation and powerlessness, consequences of stigma underpinned with stereotyping, prejudice and indifference.

The lives these men live and the stories these men tell inform the work we do.

Our philosophy is that all men are worthy of respect and their life experiences are of great value to themselves and to the group. As Maslow (1943) observed *"we are not in a position in which we have nothing to work with. We already have capacities, talents, direction, missions, and callings*".

Our emphasis is on recognising and building upon these assets both at the individual level and at the collective, moving away from positions of powerlessness, clients/consumers of services to producers and initiators of change, what we would call active citizenship.

Over the past few years the group has moved from one that was initially directed by myself to one that is fully constituted and increasingly participatory. NGMG has three volunteer workers, two of whom developed within the group. I see my role as working with people not doing things for people, I am both facilitator and guidance worker.

In the summer of 2007 the group was evaluating and discussing what we had been doing over the last quarter, what came out of the evaluation was that there was a need for some type of social activity that the men could take part in during the summer evenings and weekends that would not necessitate my attendance.

A number of scenarios were put forward one of which was to have an allotment. The rational was simple and empowering. By having an allotment we would then have somewhere the members could go any time they wanted with very little cost. It would be a place they could call their own, have BBQ's, socialise, exercise (green gym), have fun and of course grow their own food. It would be a place where the men would be able to interact with other groups and individuals, and establish connections with outside agencies.

This all seemed something that was achievable and sustainable and addressed another issue that the men had been concerned about – what would happen if we were unable to secure funding for the group in the future? Where would we go? An allotment seemed to offer possibilities.

The questions the men raised and the consequent answers they came too seemed to me to fit into current ideas around urban agriculture as a means of enabling social inclusion. The American Community Gardening Association (ACGA) articulates our objectives succinctly.

> *"Community gardening improves the quality of life for people by providing a catalyst for neighbourhood and community development, stimulating social interaction, encouraging self-reliance, beautifying neighbourhoods, producing nutritious food, reducing family food budgets, conserving resources and creating opportunities for recreation, exercise, therapy and education"* (ACGA, 2006).

Although the intention was for the men to have a place that would not necessitate my attendance I still had a role to play through facilitation and encouraging forms of organisation that were participative. I also had a role in raising member's awareness of issues they themselves would articulate through discussion, informal debates, and conversation and passing comments.

From my perspective the allotment would be a vehicle for developing opportunities around community capacity building. In the autumn of 2007 we proceeded to realise our ideas. Through local knowledge within the group we were able to identify a site that we could move into immediately, that had good transport links and where there were already various community-funded agencies that we felt we could work with.

Several of the men came down to have a look at the site; we then negotiated with the allotment secretary as to what allotment plot we were to be allocated. Many of the men voiced concerns as to how we were going to proceed. The land we had been given was very overgrown, neglected, there were old derelict buildings on it, rubble, corrugated asbestos roof tiles and glass all over the place; it looked as if it had been used as a tip.

Looking around the allotment gardens there were many plots that were in a not dissimilar state of neglect, but there were exceptions. The British Trust for Conservation Volunteers (BCTV) had an allotment and they invited us to have a look around. We could see that their plot was adequately fenced, well kept, productive and that it had made best use of local materials that had been recycled. Talking to the group worker and some of the volunteers we were persuaded that the piece of land we had could be as productive as their own, it would just take planning, commitment and time. Most importantly for us they were a group that had gone through a similar process as ourselves and we could use them as a visual example of what could be achieved and approach them for advice and support if needed.

Talking with the men over a period of time, we developed a strategy that would be flexible enough to meet the member's needs and take cognisance of changing circumstances. The strategy was simple; there would be two stages. Stage one would be developing the land so that it was suitable for production and stage two would be the actual cultivation. To enable this to happen there was a need for some form of organisation. From a community learning and development perspective seeking to enable member's empowerment, participation was paramount, so the more decentralised, horizontal and consensus seeking that form of organising was the better.

Within the group there were a number of men that had worked in the park departments, men that had joinery skills, DIY skills and those that had some experience with allotments. These were assets that could be shared and passed on to other members.

Stage one

We proceeded to:

Clear the land
Flatten the land
Fence the land (due to rabbit and deer predation)
Build a hut (for tools)
Build raised beds

This took us approximately 7 months, in that time we also had to organise weekly work parties (not all the men were able or willing to participate in the physical work), pay allotment fees, find the means of acquiring: tools, fence posts, rabbit fencing, a hut, wood for raised beds, nails, screws, timber preservative and concrete mix for fence posts.

Through our own fundraising at car boot sales and supermarket bag packing and with the support of Rosemount Lifelong Learning, Clyde Action, discounts from various retailers and timber that was donated from building sites, we were able to acquire all the items that enabled us to position ourselves where we could then move onto:

Stage two

Plant vegetables and fruit
Harvest
Prepare land for following spring

During this time several of the men took part in various horticultural courses that were provided by local agencies, North Glasgow Community Food Initiative and Lambhill Stables. This enhanced our capability and confidence, enabling us to make better use of our space. It was also an opportunity to let other agencies know what we were doing and what we were trying to achieve.

Throughout all phases of this work we would have frequent BBQ's, sit down at the allotment and go over what we were doing, what worked, didn't work, take photographs for distanced travelled and generally socialise. There was a growing interaction with some of the allotment users, the sharing of resources and information and through this an increasing awareness of issues concerning the allotments and the wider community. This increasing awareness was instrumental in moving the men away from a position off exclusivity 'this is our project' to one that recognised that our sustainability would require the sharing of ideas, resources and collective action.

There was a need to deal with issues that had a real bearing on the sustainability of the allotments. These issues the men identified as:

Vandalism
Derelict land
Lack of toilets
Fly tipping
Allotment plots not being used

We identified three reasons why we thought the situation was how it was:

The committee (not proactive and no clear strategy)
Lack of community in the allotments.
Lack of participation by the local community

Recognising these factors that we believed were pertinent enabled us to develop a strategy for change. We started to talk to some of the allotment holders about these issues, many of them were issues they had already raised with us in conversation, these we put back to them but with intention. What could we do to change the way things were. We decided that we would need representation on the committee, we looked to other allotment users to support us and through that dialogue other allotment users also decided that they would be willing to stand. While we were waiting for the community gardens committees AGM we became proactive in trying to bring about change.

- We began to clear some of the derelict land
- Mark out potential future plots
- Encourage people within the wider community to become allotment users

It was also imperative that we tried to build community within the allotments. To that end we invited all the allotment users to a bonfire/BBQ night. Only two of the plot holders participated, the men were disappointed but it was a good indicator as to how little community was in the allotments and gave us a clear idea as to where we were staring from.

Looking back on the work we have done and where we are at the moment we can reasonably say that many of our initial objectives have been met and in the process of realising these objectives we have had to develop new ones, a new vision, as we have moved away from a position of exclusivity to one of inclusivity.

If we view what we have achieved from a perspective of what we are doing as community based urban agriculture, we can then legitimately frame these achievements within its seven dimensions. This gives us a framework to deconstruct and analyse what we created.

These dimensions of community capital found within Community Based Urban Agriculture (CBUA) activities are:

- **Human Capital**: the health, education, skills of the individuals involved

- **Social Capital**: the strength of groups, networks, the common vision among their members, and the creation of bridging networks across different groups

- **Political Capital**: the dynamics of group organisation and leadership, and relations with government and supporting agencies

- **Cultural Capital**: the values and heritage of the community, and the celebration of such

- **Economic Capital**: the investments, savings, contracts and grants

- **Built Capital**: the physical settings – land, housing, other buildings, infrastructure

These dimensions are all predicated on human capital so the crux of any analysis is the question: what did we do that enabled the building of human capital to develop as it did?

Looking back at the initial evaluation and our subsequent outcomes we can see a pedagogical approach that was participatory, experiential and transformative. In Arnstein's ladder of citizen participation she says "*there is a critical difference between going through the empty ritual of participation and having the real power needed to affect the outcome of the process*" (Arnstein 1969: 216-224).

In my experience with the group I found that developing Arnstein's ideas around participation challenging. I was aware that the group was made up with men with various degrees of ability and perceptions of ability. Many of the men would defer to me. Partly this came out of some of the men's insecurities about their abilities and whether they would be capable, and partly I believe it came out of 'taken for granted' notions of organising that were inherently hierarchical.This seemed to me to be normal, and I expected it as a consequence of their life experiences that starts within patriarchy and is underpinned with an authoritarian 'common sense' education. Freire refers to this as 'banking education' where "*the learner is 'object' rather than 'subject' of the learning process*" (Mayo 1999: 59).

My approach to enabling a culture of participation was to develop consensus; seeking within the group through encouraging group discussion and asking questions. Underpinning this was a horizontal style of interaction that was in contrast to members experience of top down learning, where we were all teaching and learning from each other, where no one person was seen having all the answers. We created an environment in which people could suggest and be listened to and where their ideas could become shared actions.

Within this environment of learning, men were encouraged to take on roles and responsibilities as they became more familiar and increasingly confident of their ability to make a difference in the allotment. That difference in its most obvious form was the very landscape they worked in. Uri Gordon (2008) an anarchist theoretician talks about a primitive power that lays behind all notions of power that is the power to alter physical reality. He likens it to the Spanish word 'poder' which as a noun means 'power' and as a verb 'to be able to'. For many of the men and me, that 'power', 'being able to' was part of a transformative experience that shaped and changed perceptions of what we were capable of. As we moved from a position of segregation to integration we began to exercise that power. As Freire put it "*integration results from the capacity to adapt oneself to reality plus the capacity to make choices and to transform that reality*" (Freire 1996).

By transforming our physical reality we were able to perceive and create new realities. Looking over what we have done and how we developed one can see where practice could have been enhanced. Certainly there were different levels of participation within the group and not all the men were able to make the connections between what we were doing and how it could impact on the wider community and how that wider community was impacting on us. They may have been able to reiterate ideas; observations and thoughts that were expressed within discussion but not necessarily understand their implications.

Here there may have been opportunities for a pedagogical approach that was more focused on developing the individual's cognitive ability. In hindsight I could have involved a number of agencies from the outset and have consulted as to how we could have worked together to develop practice. It was only over time that I came to realise that there were a number of programmes and projects that could have offered advice and support from the outset.

Again I think it would have been worthwhile with the group to visit, look at and study other projects within Scotland that were using urban agriculture as a means to developing community capacity rather than making decisions as to how to proceed with very little practical knowledge. Different perspectives and ways of 'doing' enable choice and enhance the ability to make informed decisions.

Although our project has met its objectives and set new ones that are more community focused and proactive I still have concerns around its sustainability, as far as funding our project, raising money through our own endeavours will suffice. The real concern around sustainability is the ratio of physically active men that can sustain the hard work required to maintain the allotment. Many of the men that have participated are not in a position where they could take over that role if some of these members were to leave. This is something that is worth considering when developing a similar project. I have known a number of projects that have petered out due to the lack of having people that can do the hard work that is required to maintain an allotment.

This project the men took on is a place/site where many of the aims and objectives of government policy on social exclusion can be met. We see obvious benefits for a healthier Scotland, lifelong learning and employability to name but a few.

One of the inferences for government and local authorities is that this type of project can be developed with very small amounts of funding, the major barrier to this form of capacity building is access to suitable land for developing into allotments – always an issue as waiting lists for allotments in Glasgow and Scotland in general are at record highs.

In conclusion through our project and the development of practice we have come to understand that the use of allotments within local communities can have great relevance as a media for therapy, as a mechanism for social inclusion and for the development of community capital.

Ambra Burls, a senior lecturer and researcher in Mental Health at Anglia Ruskin University's Institute of Health and Social Care says in his paper *Ecotherapy in Practice and Education* (2004) that the benefits of interaction with nature for the general population is more pronounced in people with disabilities and those who are socially marginalized. His research implies that their wellbeing is demonstrably improved and they are less socially excluded when they interact with nature. He goes onto to say that "*they also reconnect with their communities, some reaching a higher level of socio-political identity".*

Certainly for the men's group the benefit of working within the allotment has had obvious therapeutic value that has enabled various social dimensions to develop, in particular men were constantly changing roles within the group, at one moment they were teaching and at another they were learning, some were becoming links to other allotment users and the wider community and others were becoming activists, initiators of change that has culminated in one of our members being elected onto the allotment committee and with our support the election of a number of other allotment users with similar ideas as our own.

Working together as a team in the allotment has been an enjoyable, life enriching experience that has had pervasive effects for all the participants, for some it has been transformative.

Commentary

Working with men is often a difficult area for development work. Women's group are often seen as easy to organise and more productive as women are more likely to take on developmental issues.

This study discusses some of the issue of working with men. It explores the value of gardening based projects (an underdeveloped area of potential for community activity). These activities are then explored in relation to wellbeing and the creation of human capital.

Practice Study 6

Women's Group

Sarah Jane McNeil

Abstract

This study is set in the context of a local trust developing a range of programmes on employability, care and regeneration activities. From these activities a women's group is established.

The Study

Inverclyde is a local authority area in the West of Scotland with a population of around 80,000 inhabitants. It is known for its high levels of deprivation and alcohol abuse, and according to the Chartered Society of Physiotherapy, it has one of the lowest life expectancy rates in not only Scotland, but Britain too. But at the heart of this once industrial thriving town, is an organisation that keeps working away to build the people of Inverclyde up and provide opportunity's that they otherwise wouldn't get.

Inverclyde Community Development Trust is one of the biggest voluntary organisations in Scotland. The Trust, as it is known, has been going strong for 23 years, changing shape with the needs of the communities that it works in. The Trust is currently government funded, which often meant its projects often changed, due to funding requirements. This study focuses on developmental work for the Trust with a local women's group.

The Trust

Inverclyde Community Development Trust has 3 main sections.

- Trust Care Services
- Trust Employability Services
- Trust Regeneration Services

These are then broken down again further with different projects and services being provided within each one.

The organisation is currently reviewing their services and is looking at how they are engaging with the people in their communities. In recent years their focus has been on employability within Inverclyde, which had a huge influence on the services of the Trust. They are keen to bring community development back into the Trust, and my purpose was to pilot a piece of work that would link Trust Employability Services to the Volunteer Centre Inverclyde (another project of the Trust). The Trust offered an integrated service, but the links weren't always that straight forward. The Organisation has access to the community on a daily basis through the number of services they have and the programmes they put on, but were guilty of overlooking their client's true needs. They often attended programmes then went back to their normal lives with no aftercare service or no option to progress onto somewhere else. The Trust were looking for me to engage in a listening survey with their clients and find any common interests that they shared that they may then want to meet voluntary as a group to explore. They were hoping this would potentially give the clients the opportunity to stay together as volunteers and explore community based themes together.

Paulo Freire was according to Ledwith, "*proven to be one of the outstanding visionary thinkers of our time in the field of education for freedom*" (1997:61). Freire used Popular Education techniques with his emphasis on dialogue and his concern for the oppressed. Through *'dialogue'* he felt that you came to the *concept of praxis – reflection and action.* As Freire's work had made a big impact on my own learning, taking me from a magical consciousness to a critical one, I felt that this was the model that I wanted to use with my group.

This would be a new and exciting challenge for me. Although I was still within the confines of the organisation that I work for as a youth worker, this opportunity would let me stretch myself. In my practice, I was very guilty of only working with young people. The nature of the work would allow me to come away from my normal environment, stretching my comfort zone, and experience a new way of working.

For the first part of work I was asked to sit in on several training courses that Trust Employability staff were putting on for clients. These courses were both open to New Deal Clients (mandatory) and anyone in the community who wished to sign up to these. These courses were held at both in-house at the Port Glasgow Business and Training Centre, but also out in the 'Hubs' (community centres).

I sat in an assertiveness course facilitated by one of the Trust's programme workers. I joined in with the group rather than sitting on the side line observing. I felt that this would be a better way to *'listen'* to the group. I didn't want to make myself an outsider and make them feel if I was watching them in some way. I wanted to be part of their process. I wanted us to *'work and learn together'* I felt that by doing this, they would gain my trust, and I would be able to share their hopes and fears.

This was the point when I first got to listen to the clients. As the course did have both mandatory and voluntary clients on it there was mixed feelings. I could hear the frustrations of the New Deal clients. They were on a 13 week course to get them ready for work. The Trust had recently changed the course from a 13 week job search programme to a 13 week programme full of options that where provided by the programme workers of the Trust. They could choose from a number of 2 week options to one day courses. Anything from trade skills, to assertiveness sessions were on offer. This had been a well thought out process from the Trust's behalf. They wanted to equip the people being made to come on this 13 week mandatory course with skills they could use for life and tasters that may introduce them to a possible career.

But the clients were telling me that they felt as *"if the Trust had no clue what they were doing and were just sending them anywhere to fill their time."* I found myself sticking up for the organisation as I genuinely felt that they were trying to provide the best service and opportunities that they could for their clients. I felt that the Trust were also working here to the National Occupational Standards practice principles here too, in the best way that they could within the confines of their funding. I felt the Trust was trying to make clients more self–determined.

I tried to explain the organisations choices as best as I could to the clients, It fell on deaf ears. After a while I just listened intently to their fears. They had nothing against us as workers but felt that they were not given any choice in whether they participated or not. I started to question these people's real needs? This made me think of Maslow's hierarchy of needs. Maslow (1943) argued that people were only motivated if their basic needs were being met. If these people's needs were not being met, why would they ever want to come back as a voluntary group? I started to realise that achieving work objectives wasn't going to be as easy as I first had hoped.

Another group that I sat in on was an 8 week Skills for Confidence course. The course ran 3 days a week and was aimed at women to build upon their confidence, not only for their personal lives, but also for getting ready to get back to work. The group was a mixture of both mandatory clients (New Deal Programme) and voluntary clients referred from Trust Employability Services. I sat in on the group at various intervals throughout their 8 weeks to get to know the women and gain their trust. I had planned to use popular education techniques with them. I would start off by listening and this would then give me the basis to move on to presenting a *code* back to the group.

Through listening to them, I was realising that they were anxious about the course coming to an end and was keen to stay together as they have built relationships with each other. Each of the women had their own issues and was there for their own reasons, but the main being they lacked in confidence. Over the 8 weeks I could see how the group were forming, and building trust with each other. They also had trust with me and when giving them the possibility of staying together, with me supporting that, they jumped at the chance.

As a worker, this also scared me a little. A women's group was something I never thought I would work with, and if to be really honest, never wanted to. This made me look at my values and question where this feeling was coming from. Should I not be inclusive, non-judgemental? I realised that I felt that I would have nothing to offer them. That they were real women with real lived experiences far more varied and interesting than my own. I was still a young woman, who lived at home, never experienced motherhood, nor confidence issues. All in all I feel I have had a privileged life. I felt a little overwhelmed by it all. How could I support this group to plan for change and take some sort of collective action?

I felt I had to speak to my supervisor, to let her know how I was feeling. We decided that since the women had shown an interest in the Arts and Crafts course, we would offer this to them after they finished the confidence course. This would give me the opportunity to listen further. David Gauntlett in his book Making and Connecting Agenda suggests that *"through making things, and sharing them with others, we increase our engagement with the world"* (2007). He goes on to discuss the idea that when people are engaged in making things their "*brains are can be open to new perspectives, and reflecting upon things we have made can suggest new ideas and ways of doing things."* I wanted to the women to be exploring things as they were creating.

As I was leading the course, I could choose what we were creating. I chose to start off with an Art Journal, to start them on their journey of reflection.

The group did start reflecting on the first week of the Arts and Crafts course. I was aware that there was a lot of the personal coming up in discussion. I acknowledge that this would be a natural progression for the women as they had gained trust with each other and were keen to share their historic narratives. Ledwith in Community Development: A Critical Approach discusses the individual level:

> *"The individual level is the foundation of our work. It is the level at which we anchor what we do in the lived realities of the people with whom we work, and which gives relevance to our work in their lives. Individual stories become collective narratives that express hopes and fears, needs and strengths that are the basis of theory and practice."*

I could feel these women's hopes and fears. Many didn't want to "*go back to the place they had been*" before their confidence course and the admitted that they weren't ready to leave each other either. I thought that this would be an ideal time to approach the subject of staying together and how this would look. After discussing this with the group, they were really excited and pleased that they would be staying together as a group. I knew it was a little rushed, and it was only a small piece of action, but I felt that this was the ideal opportunity to get the ball rolling and take the first steps to supporting the group to *identify aims and objectives for collective action.*

On the day the group participated well. The group had never done anything like this before and since only 3 turned up, I kept it quite informal according to the groups needs. We decided that the next week, when we were meeting for the first time as volunteers, we would explore aims and objectives more fully. I had planned a session around this using the Training for Transformation books (Hope and Timmel 1995). I hoped to eventually get them to be looking at local and global issues and to be exploring the world around them. I also wanted them to start planning how we could open up the group to more women. At this point I felt that I was adhering to the practice principles of the NOS, especially *Reflective Practice and Self Determination.* Although we weren't monitoring and evaluating our time together formally, we had made a Blossom Tree and the women where writing their reflections of the day and putting them onto the tree. I feel I was being open to the groups needs, and rearranging or putting aside my session plans when something else in the group came up.

The next week though and the next few sessions after, the group weren't keen to move on. Some members of the group were just happy to stay as they were and be provided a service, even though I had explained that they would be volunteers and how the group would look and the things that they choose to do would be up to them. I had made them fully aware that I was only with them for another eight weeks. By that time hopefully they would be able to support themselves. Some of the group understood this, but others seemed unwilling to let go. Even when I put on sessions for them or asked other workers in to work with the women they couldn't get passed the personal issues to look at the wider community.

Looking back and reflecting, I rushed my group. I should have identified from the personal issues coming out that the women had needs that were not being met. This was becoming more and more apparent as the weeks went on. The group weren't moving any further on.

I was frustrated and felt that I had failed as a worker. Why couldn't I make these women move on? I went to my supervisor and discussed this with her. She assured me that it wasn't what I was doing and told me to go back and look at the Training for Transformation books that I had been consulting with. She spoke of the cycle for *Reflection and Action model.* (Hope and Timmel 2003:21). As soon as she mentioned this, I felt relieved.

We then went on to discuss why it is so important to link theory to your practice. Not to let you off the hook as such, but to understand the process and what is happening. This will allow you to look objectively at the situation. It took me right out of the situation and to understand what was happening. I also used my group work theory here too, using Tuckman's model (1965) to realise that the group were in a constant state of forming. This made it hard for me to get to the evaluating and monitoring process. The group were in a constant process of starting, going around and around in a cycle and I was getting frustrated; frustrated that the timescale of the work was making me want to push these women along even though I knew they weren't ready. How could I get the group to move on if they weren't ready? I found that as a worker, you are often in conflict with yourself and the others around you.

I felt I had suffocated myself, I had been too organised and was rushing in with community sessions that the group weren't interested in participating in. I was also in conflict with the group, whom I felt at times were in a *magical consciousness*. I wanted this to be a natural progression, I wanted to move along at the pace of the group, but these other factors were making me *shape* the group as such. I wondered if this was what they were truly looking for, or was I unconsciously pulling them the way I wanted it to go? I questioned whether there was such a thing as true community development? I acknowledge that if this was my job and I was getting paid, then I would also be feeling this conflict due to the constraints of funding. If you are a paid worker sent in to do a job with a group then, it isn't pure community development. As long as you adhere to the standards and your values and principles and take a community development approach, then you could make it as pure as it would ever get.

I wondered where the women's group sat in this structure. If it wasn't pure community development and it wasn't service delivery, then where did it sit? I realised that within my job as a youth worker, at times I had been *tokenistic* and put on things that I felt that young people had needed and not what they had expressed themselves. I had the power, and didn't realise I was using it. Although this time, through *reflective practice*, I was more than aware that the women were handing the power over to me and this felt really uncomfortable. I kept trying to explain that the group was all about them, but they were still keen to just follow my lead.

Drysdale and Purcell (2001) ask the question, in relation to the power that exists in a partnership when implementing participation on a course of action, *"...do we all decide equally or do some people have more influence in decision making than others?"* As equality was one of my values, this was sitting uncomfortably with me. Is there such a thing as equality? How can you treat everyone equally when some have more needs than others? I came to the realisation that it was OK to have a little more power, as the group wouldn't move on if I didn't make the decisions sometimes. It still didn't feel right though, but was that not my job as a community worker? To support groups to develop a plan of collective action? I had to really ask myself, was this really what the group wanted or needed? I felt tired and frustrated and wondered if it was me that was holding the group back? Were they pushing themselves in order to satisfy me? Were they just going along with the ride, happy in the knowledge that they have somewhere to go every week? The group were *participating* but were they really getting to the self –determination point? At the bottom of Shelly Arnstein's (1969) Ladder of Participation is manipulation. Was I manipulating them with my own agenda? How could I empower them? Should I empower them?

Evans (1992) highlights the paradox created by acknowledging that *"there is a basic contradiction in the idea of people empowering others because the very institutional structure that puts one group in a position to empower also works to undermine the act of empowerment."* I can see how workers often abuse their power and disempower communities, creating a dependency to keep them in a job. Also, the funding that is allocated to communities often comes from the Government, whom have their own agenda. I had to question whether the Trust wanted to fill this gap that they had, just to be able to apply more funding. If we found a need for a women's group, would this make the Trust in a better position to receive more money? To be honest, I know this wasn't the Trusts intention in this case but often organisations and projects are guilty of this, often changing shape to suit the criteria of the newest government initiative.

The values that I had made this feel uncomfortable to me. Do the people that make the decisions ever truly consult with the communities that they make the decisions for? How do you deal with that as a worker?

Eventually, I had to be honest with the group and ask them if this was what they truly wanted. I felt that I had achieved the group to take action but that I was struggling to get them to evaluate anything. They were constantly going around in *the reflection - action cycle* but not really getting anywhere.

After an incident with one of the women, I had to be honest with her and explain that the group wasn't what she needed, that it was another service. After this the group eventually moved on. The group are holding a Tea Party to ask other women in. They are also making a booklet on Local Women who have made a difference to their community I now acknowledge that community work is a slow process, often very demanding of a worker's energy. It can be stressful too for a worker, especially one who needs to meet outcomes and objectives.

I got more out of the women's group than I could ever have hoped to imagine. We may not have taken a big piece of action, but in relation to my practice, the women have been the biggest action in all of my learning. They are the ones who kicked me out of my comfort zone and made me deal with situations that normally I would avoid or shy away from. They are the ones that put me in a position that made me question my values, question my organisation and question myself.

They opened up their lives to me and gave me a perspective on being women that I hadn't been privy to before. We laughed, we cried but most of all we shared. *"Community workers are privileged to be accepted into people's lives in the community and with this privilege comes a responsibility to develop relationships that are mutual, reciprocal, dignified and respectful. These underlying values emerge from an ideology of equality, and they shape every aspect of our practice, determining the way that we plan and conduct specific projects."* (Ledwith 2005:32)

I look back and realise that I shouldn't have been worried about I could give them. *Working and learning* together is all about participation and exactly what it says on the tin, Working and Learning together. This was what we were achieving as a group. We may not have been making big giant steps, but sometimes change is more lasting when taking one small step at a time

Commentary

This study is very reflective with the worker constantly checking the nature and progress of the work against her value set. She also questions the effect of state funding has on the shape of community development practice.

Within the discussion of practice within the women's group a range of questions are explored including the way group objectives are decided, relative power relationships, the time a group needs to develop and the pressure from agencies to move it along. This discussion is related to ideas around empowerment and Freire's reflection-vision-planning-action cycle.

Practice Study 7

Sikh women and their families

Trishna Sing

Abstract

This study explores a community health initiative for Sikh women. It is an example of partnership working between the NHS and a community based organisation. The motive for the work was to implement the local NHS health promotion agenda. However, it also created a range of developmental opportunities for the community organisation.

The Study

Sikh Sanjog was set up in 1989 and seeks to addresses the unmet needs of Sikh women and their families living in Leith Edinburgh. Leith is a mixed community where approximately one hundred and fifty Sikh families live. Lothian Borders has a Minority Ethnic population of 2.8% around 21,800 people (Census 2000).

Most of the Leith Sikhs are Bhatra Sikhs, who were traditionally a vendor class; in the Punjab they were mainly selling wares door-to-door, small shopkeepers and expert fortune-tellers. They mostly came from the Punjab, which eventually became the state of Pakistan following independence from British Rule in1947. However this has changed recently with a large number of Sikhs from other communities and overseas students moving into the area. Overall the majority of Sikhs still in Leith are still from the Bhatra community.

The first generation of Bhatra Sikh women born in the UK were raised in exactly the same way as though they were living in the India of 1947. This was mainly due to the fact that their parents and grandparents were and in some instances still are, living within the cultural boundaries of the village lifestyle of the Indian that they left behind in 1947. Restrictions on education and social activities have been placed on the majority of the females from this particular community throughout their lives.

The main aim of the project was to work in partnership with the communities' values and provide a confidential service. To do this, the project employs an outreach development worker who is from the community and encourages the project team to respond to the communities concerns.

With this in mind, the structure of the organisation reflects its aims to support the Sikh women, as half its staff and volunteers are from within the Sikh community. Similarly the Management Committee was made up of volunteers, who are service users and professionals from a variety of agencies including Community Education, advisory agencies such as Citizen' and Social Work.

Sikh Sanjog provides a range of quality opportunities for Sikh women and their families in response to educational, recreational, cultural, and social needs, recognising the potential for life-long learning, social and economic inclusion. Promoting links between Sikhs and the wider communities it is a stepping-stone for women to access mainstream resources and services.

As an example of 'partnership working' I will be looking in detail at the Women's Walking Group which was a health initiative the main aim was to promote healthy hearts and healthy living.

> "*Health Promotion – By encompassing education, health improvement, the reduction of health inequalities and community development – seeks to make real the desire to improve the health status of a defined population through a series of targeted actions taken in concert with other agencies, voluntary organisations and the public*" (Bhopal et. Al. 2002)

The focus of the pilot project was to look at the high rate of coronary heart disease and diabetes in the South Asian population. In line with government policy, current priority areas for action within the North East Edinburgh local Health Care Co-operative comprised of improved health care for ethnic minority communities with targeted services in respect of coronary heart disease and diabetes. The aim was to set up a pilot project wherein a dedicated clinic would be set up offering local South Asian people screening and risk assessment in respect of coronary heart disease and diabetes.

For example research has shown (Lothian NHS 2008) that coronary heart disease, strokes, cancer, and accidents are among the main causes of death in all groups. Diabetes however is three to four times more common in Indians, Pakistanis, and Bangladeshis than in the population as a whole. Services need to be aware of disease patterns and while there is no need for separate services, the process of service delivery may need to be adapted to be effective. Addressing the health needs of minority ethnic women has not generally been included as an integral part of past planning processes, but has been based on specific initiatives and project-based work.

Central Leith is home to around 2000 Asians and it was therefore agreed that a small team of workers should explore the local situation to assess whether or not current health provisions were adequately meeting the needs in respect of coronary heart disease and diabetes services.

The aim was to set up a pilot project wherein a dedicated clinic would be set up offering local South Asian people screening and risk assessment in respect of coronary heart disease and diabetes. The initial working group would comprise of two members of the LHCC Health Inequalities Group and key representatives from the various south Asian communities. A steering group would be formed for the duration of the project i.e. May 2002 – June 2003. The ultimate goal of the project was to keep in line with NHS Lothian's "*commitment to work towards mainstreaming racial equality in all policies and practices through signing the Rooting out Racism declaration*" (Lothian NHS. 2008).

The responsibilities of the community representatives would be to act as liaison between the Steering Group, project workers and members of their respective communities. To provide information and feedback from the communities who may wish to become involved in leading future project activities. Furthermore, a training programme was put into action covering the topics of Introduction to Coronary Heart Disease, Diabetes, Basic Life Support, Jogging, Nutrition and a Walking programme. This was offered to the community workers to raise their awareness of these issues, so they would be better informed themselves before taking it to the communities. Unfortunately the health professionals seemed to think that after only one or two day training programmes, we were qualified enough to hold training days for our respective communities.

Despite these hiccups the Clinic opened on a weekly basis, with alternative days for male and female screenings and at the same time co-ordinating a series of healthy lifestyle activities e.g. exercise classes, healthy eating workshops and a walking programme to provide graded low level exercise that most people could participate in safely. The idea was that one or two of the local community members would be willing to undertake the appropriate training and take it back to their groups. Sikh Sanjog felt that the walking course would be ideal for us; it was something that we would be able to encourage our women to take part in on a weekly basis. The aim of our Walking Group was to encourage the women:

- To change their sedentary lifestyles
- To highlight the benefits of walking to them
- To reduce their isolation.

The objective was to equip them with the confidence to enable them to select the best options that would benefit them and their families. In relation to health issues the aim was:

- To supply them with meaningful health information, that they could apply to their own lifestyles.
- To encourage them to access mainstream health care.

To promote the Walking Group we held an Open Day inviting all our members. In total 30 Sikh women attended the event. We highlighted the benefits of walking by way of one-to-one talks and group discussions. The main point was to inform everyone that "*the biggest health improvements are gained by encouraging inactive people to do a modest amount of exercise. Brisk walking is the ideal form of exercise to achieve this progression and so maintain good physical health*" (Blair 1989). In the initial 2-3 weeks of the Walking Group we put our training to use by informing the women of the benefits of walking:

- It was free
- Required no special equipment or expense
- Is accessible to everyone regardless of age, ability or income
- Can be enjoyed safely
- Can be incorporated into daily routine easily
- Regular exercise can reduce blood pressure

- Reduces cholesterol
- Helps prevent Type 2 diabetes
- Benefits immune system, proves muscle strength
- Reduces anxiety and depression

Overall they would lose weight! (AMA)

The Walking Group started in September 2002 and our route was from the Sikh Sanjog office to the local park. Our target was to walk for 45 minutes with 15 minutes warm up, registration, and allowing for latecomers. In the first five weeks we did one circuit of the park, gradually building up over the next five weeks to two circuits – still keeping within our time of 45 minutes.

By the end of the first three months we held an open discussion with the group to evaluate and see if we had fulfilled some of the aims and objectives we had set for ourselves. The comments were as follows:

- Feeling more active
- Less depressed
- Less aches and pains
- Motivation to lose weight
- Less feeling of isolation
- More secure to discuss personal problems with each other

For example many of the women faced problems with in-laws and some of the women had problems with daughter- in- laws there were some who were living with alcohol abuse and financial problems. All of these subjects seemed like taboo too talk about when they met at the Sikh Gurdwara (temple) as this is the main meeting place of the whole community so pleasantries are exchanged and people never really get the chance to talk.

There is the stigma that is attached to your standing in the community that prevents women from discussing any subject like this unless it is with a member of the family in some cases even discussing it within the family becomes impossible. Although the walking group was open to anyone our group consisted of all Sikh women this gave them the opportunity to discuss some of the subjects I have mentioned, when talking amongst themselves there came the gradual realisation that they were not alone with their problems. Confidentiality became the key for this group and allowed them a space to take strength from each other and cope with their problems.

As an agency it gave us an opening to bring a variety of agencies that could help deal with some of these problems thus opening up other avenues of support that otherwise would never have been accessed by this group e.g. Libra (organisation that works with women affected by alcohol issues) Cruse Bereavement.

Furthermore the women had started to walk from their homes to the office instead of getting lifts in cars. They encouraged each other, and also told other members of the community how it had helped them and so brought new members to join the group. One woman lost at least three stone gradually over the two-year period that the Walking Group has been established. In her own words:

> "*Walking made me feel good, and I wanted to lose weight. With encouragement from the walk leaders I joined the keep-fit class and swimming group. I know I would not have been able to do this on my own. It was the walking that started me off.*"

We learned a lot about health issues and welcomed the opportunity to develop these further. We already had the skills and potential in facilitating and running groups and so when training was offered to become keep fit instructors we encouraged one of our group member to apply for the post. She took part in a 26-week programme at college fully supported by Sikh Sanjog at all times. This included educational, moral and financial support i.e. travel expenses. Throughout this she continued as a volunteer walk leader. This gave her experience to facilitate her future keep-fit classes and she is now a qualified keep-fit instructor and lay Health Worker with the local Health Care Co-operative.

Being bi-lingual means that she can continue to encourage ethnic minority women to access these classes. Sometimes language can be a great barrier for these women explaining the benefits of exercise in their own language takes on a different perspective for them. By encouraging this woman and providing the one-to-one support she needed to enable her to go on the course and complete it, we felt we were working alongside the NHS to achieve their aim "*to ensure that the employment policies and practices of all parts of the NHS in*

Lothian do not discriminate against minority ethnic communities and do promote equal opportunities. To work toward creating and maintaining a workforce that reflects the diversity of communities in Edinburgh and Lothian's. This may involve the use of positive action as allowed under legislation, where there is under-representation of staff from minority ethnic communities" (Lothian NHS)

Although we feel that the project has been an overall success, there were many major problems that arose through lack of communication between the NHS staff and ourselves. At the outset of the project we were given the impression that this would be a coalition of our work. We were led to believe that we would be paid sessional hours as most of us worked part-time. Although all this had been discussed in detail with the NHS workers when they were applying for the funding, it emerged that they had been required to apply to a separate 'pot' of funding to pay sessional workers. This had been unsuccessful but they had withheld this information and put forward the idea of payment 'in-kind' i.e. the training programmes that we had participated in would normally have been paid for by our projects through the NHS.

We had put it to them that our part in the project needed to be valued, as we had the experience and understanding of our community. We were well established in the area, and over the years we had built trust and co-operation with the community. As a community group we were closely in touch with our interest group and any developing situations. We would be able to identify and respond to changing needs more quickly than the statutory sector.

Therefore "*communication between health professionals and service users was key to the success of this initiative. There was a need to provide effective transmission of health messages through a variety of culturally sensitive means. These included providing forums for open discussion in safe and familiar settings, conducting workshops, employing bi-lingual workers, disseminating translated materials and identified areas of concern, conducting outreach work and liaising with Minority Ethnic Agencies*" (Bhatnagar and Ines 1994)

Many aspects of the provision of healthcare need to be improved both in terms of cultural sensitivity and any elements that would be seen as racist in specific areas, like the provision of food, a choice of gender of health professionals and interpreters.

There then came a gradual realisation amongst ourselves including the line manager that we were being used by this professional team. We were the bridge that they had used to reach a really 'difficult to reach community'. We were made to feel grateful for the training that had been provided for us by the project, and that we had an obligation to fulfil the roles of the link-workers. It would have been a disservice to our client group if we had opted out of this venture, as many organisations and individuals did due solely to the fact that they realised early on that the NHS was using them in a tokenistic way.

The inability of state welfare to respond to the needs of minority groups without being tokenistic is a reflection of its failure to offer them opportunities to participate adequately in important decision making mechanisms and shape the way services are delivered. Furthermore this small project highlighted the fact that funding streams to autonomous BME organisations remain marginal within most large-scale mainstream policy initiatives. (Craig et al 2005, Craig 2006).

In hindsight we realised we should have had more time to familiarise ourselves with the way that the NHS structure operates. The NHS had no idea of how the voluntary sector operate, i.e. the flexibility and openness that is required to make organisations like ours successful in reaching a client group. In future we would follow the guidelines written down in the Scottish Compact Good Practice Guide:

> *"Identify at the outset the contribution each partner is expected to make. Clarify whether expenses will be paid to small organisations. Identify what happens if agreement cannot be reached and a partner wishes to withdraw; and be aware that effective voluntary sector participation involves costs. Agree suitable methods for ongoing dialogue to facilitate contributions to policy and implementation.*" (Scottish Compact Good Practice Guide)

We have all gained a greater awareness of our position in society as women. When the women in the group got to know each other, and started sharing their experiences of health problems it opened other issues that affected their lives. Taking part in the discussion groups has given them the confidence to face and challenge some of the internal barriers including the gender bias that is prevalent in many Sikh families.

I feel that health has been a good starting point for the women to get involved in the community action; it is a subject that is relevant to all women in addition to the roles we are encouraged to take on i.e. wife, mother, daughter, etc. A woman's health is something of which she is very aware having suffered, sometimes quite considerably, through inappropriate care from the health service. The absence of anyone with whom to share anxieties, many women will welcome an opportunity to talk about their health and well-being.

Having gained confidence from each other's support the women have more control over their own health and are more able to confront attitudes within the health service and other areas that affect their lives. They became able to demand a type of provision or service that is suitable to their needs and culture. The desire to move on from where we are also provides the impetus to acquire new knowledge and skills. With this in mind, a number of Sikh women have trained as interpreters for the N.H.S.

However, in different ways community can be the space that women struggle to define as theirs. Whether it is for health facilities that are responsive to their needs, for better housing, transport, for freedom from sexual and/or racial harassment. For non-racist, non-sexist child care provision. For equal training and employment opportunities, the space to celebrate and not hide their sexuality or ethnicity.

Commentary

This is a good example of the value adding potential that came come from a specific and focussed piece of work. The impetus comes from a top down health analysis of the local Asian community. The agenda was that of the NHS and the community organisation with its close links to the Asian community; the ideal vehicle to implement these policy objectives.

The study draws out some of the practice issues of such partnerships: whose agenda, whose resources, who makes the key decisions and so on? What is very useful here is the opportunities this work created for the community organisation to engage Asian women in discussions and activities that otherwise would not have taken place. From this new understandings of everyday life and associated issues emerge. Part of this process is the personal development and opportunities for people to reflect on their lives and to become involved in other activities.

It is often the case with projects like this that the real and sustained community benefit comes not from the initial project but the developmental opportunities that are created.

Practice Study 8

Grandparents Parenting Again

Carole Dick

Abstract

This practice study discusses the experiences of grandparents who are operating as 'kinship carers'. It explores issues around family self help, the vagaries of social policy and local authority services. The work was underpinned by a creative mix of Paulo Freire's ideas as a learning process within a campaigning context drawn from Saul Alinsky.

The Study

If 'sixty is the new forty' should it be a surprise that many older people are called upon to be sole cares for grandchildren? This phenomenon is being termed 'Parenting Again' by sociologists. However unlike parents and foster cares, there is no financial assistance and no provision within social policy for financial help to Grandparents Parenting Again. It is a matter of justice that Grandparents as sole carers be treated equally to other carers. In this chapter I am describing how a group of Grandparents, Parenting Again decided to challenge social policy in regard to the lack of financial help to them.

The lesson learned from this project was that people are capable of a lot more than they often think or imagine, especially with appropriate support, encouragement and help.

In this twenty first century where the *"...postmodern world is seeing a breakdown of clear age bands ,and that chronological age patterns are becoming less crucial to peoples lives..."* Macionis & Plummer (2005: 342). Community Development has an important role in working with this social group that is the subject of this study.

Politicians responsible for social policies have a difficult job as the issues raised by Parenting Again can be very complicated and are often more to do with economics than people. Social theorists and well informed community workers can help make sense of the problems and encourage communities to ask difficult questions and take proactive action in a truly Freirean way.

Well trained community workers also take risks and experiment with new ideas. I agree with Purcell (2005) who makes the point that community workers need to have an understanding of the local culture of the community they are working with to be effective workers and Alinsky (1971) in a similar vein advices community organisers to stay inside the experience of the people they are working with.

Midlothian Sure Start together with, Healthy Living Partnership Project (HELPP) and the Integration team, through joint research identified gap in service provision for Grandparents who were now sole carers for their Grandchildren within Midlothian. To address this gap a joint project between Midlothian Sure Start and Healthy Living Partnership Project was suggested. As it was initially thought family support and health related issues may be among the problems facing Grandparents who are now parenting again. I was asked if I along with the development worker from HELPP would be interested in doing a pilot project following the research.

The first step we took was to try to discover the needs of and issues facing Grandparents. I wanted to approach this from a reflective perspective, in that I felt to understand the real issues facing the Grandparents and how best to support them, we needed to listen to their stories. Inspired by Barrent–Lennard (1998) to be receptive to the whole of other people's experiences within the group as well as to listen sensitively, a relaxed atmosphere, over a cup of coffee was created. We encouraged the Grandparents to talk, allowing people to express their concerns in their own time, telling us how they had now become sole carers for their grandchildren and in one case great-grandchildren. Some of the stories were heartbreaking, mostly drug related. Along with having to cope with parenting again, there was among many of them a sense of guilt, because they blamed themselves for their children's plight.

What was becoming clear from listening to the Grandparents was what Freire (1996) describes a 'culture of silence'. The Grandparents were feeling alienated and not being heard by the dominant people in society (social services, politicians, councils). In effect the Grandparents were 'oppressed', especially so given their negative feelings about themselves and their sense of failure as parents. It became clear from listening to the Grandparents that they were emotional and angry about the lack of help from they were receiving from the social services, particularly financial help. Much as Freire (1996) explains what helped fuel their anger, was that the grandparents were in 'magical consciousnesses' where they did not know their rights so accepted the lack of help as that was how it was or *"...they still... (clung) to the old values in the simple hope that everything... (would) work out somehow, some way..."* (Alinsky 1971, p.g.xvi).

The objective for us as workers was to help break that culture of silence. To achieve this the Grandparents needed to tell their stories (the code) to other groups and to reflect on these stories. So it was arranged to visit other Grandparents out with Midlothian who were parenting again and for them to share their stories. As the Grandparents began to reflect on their similar stories, it became clear that the 'generative theme' was lack of financial helped available. Through this reflection the Grandparents moved into 'naïve consciousness' where they began to make the connection between the social, economical and political issues they were experiencing. This connection enabled the Grandparents to move to a 'critical consciousness' as Freire (1996) describes it, where they realised the issues they were facing were public issues and they needed to be heard.

Shor and Freire (1987) writing about liberation education suggest that collectively *learners* (in this case Grandparents) and *teachers* (in this case my colleague and I) through dialogue should seek to find ways of challenging the status-quo. As teachers we decided to do something collectively, instead of speaking on the Grandparents behalf to the authorities. Engaging the Grandparents in dialogue, as Shor and Freire suggest, was a means of getting the grandparents to see that they did not need to adapt themselves to the fact that there was no help. They could challenge the existing social policies and legislation, regarding grandparent's rights and responsibilities for looking after their grandchildren, together.

As this dialogue was likely to be quite hard going, we recognised that needed to get the Grandparents engaged in a creative and fun dialogue in which the participants could to feel comfortable and supported in such a way that would encourage everyone to participate. As the facilitator I was determined not to tell them how to do it, I wanted them to discover for themselves what their learning needs were and that it was possible for them to challenge the existing social policy concerning grandparents parenting again.

It was decided that 'learning circles' would be the most appropriate technique as "*...learning circles seek to be free spaces where open discussion of hard questions can take place in a collaborative and enriching environment that brings together people from different constituencies...*" quoted in Purcell (2005: 219). As Grandparents were coming from all over Midlothian learning circles would allow us to explore and discover together what the learning needs were.

The grandparents divided themselves into two groups. They were encouraged to discuss the questions: What did they think the government and local authorities could do to help? What were the needs? So that the group would not look to me, or my colleague, to start the discussion we left them to go and make the coffee, only rejoining them when we brought the coffee in. The grandparents engaged in heated discussions over the discrimination towards family caring for family they felt they were experiencing from the Social Services.

An example of such perceived discrimination was that grandparents can apply to become foster cares or to adopt, but have no guarantee that they will be allocated the grandchildren that they are already looking after. This is exacerbated by the fact that their grandchildren would be taken into care while the grandparent's applications are being processed. In some cases grandparents have been turned down because they have been deemed too old and on occasion in another local authority area, a grandmother was refused as a foster carer because she was considered to be overweight!

The grandparents felt they were also discriminated against financially by existing social policy as there was no provision for financial help for grandparents looking after their grandchildren, despite the financial sacrifices grandparents in this position have often to make. Other carers including family members are often helped financially e.g. those looking after the disabled.

The Children (Scotland) Act 1995 states local authorities have a duty to ensure *"... the positive promotion of children's welfare..."*. The Act also states that: *"help for families should be geared towards supporting the care of children in their family and community..."* However in section 22 of Children (Scotland) Act 1995 it is stated that children in care *may* be supported by cash payments. This word may appears to be open to interpretation. Local authorities have in the main chosen to use the definitions of foster care in section 50 of the Children

(Scotland) 1995 Act, as exempting Grandparents from eligibility for financial help as they are blood relatives and not 'employed' to look after their grandchildren.

As there were so many resultant definitions of what constituted Kinship Care within legislation, and no standardised policy on Kinship Care in Britain, some local authorities opted to ignore grandparents Parenting Again. For example one grandparent asked for financial help with clothing, particularly school clothing and was told that if they could not afford to keep their grandchildren then the children would be better of 'in care' elsewhere.

After much debate the grandparents put together a list of their main needs:

- Legal advice
- Financial assistance and advice
- Support and training in their changing roles
- To discover if there was any provision for grandparents as sole carers of their grandchildren in England.
- To look at ways of challenging politicians, councillors and social services in respect of lack of help for the grandparents who are 'parenting again'.

We agreed to organise a family lawyer to come and speak to the grandparents on what existing parental rights they had and how to go about demanding those rights. We invited the Welfare Rights agency to come and discuss what benefits the grandparents may be entitled to. The primary concern of the grandparents was to highlight the lack of financial provision in social policy and legislation to the politicians and councillors.

> *"Change comes from power, and power comes from organisation. In order to act people must come together...the organiser knows... that his biggest job is to give the people the feeling they can do something...to build confidence and hope in the idea of organisation and thus the people themselves..."* (Alinsky 1971: 113-114).

With shades of Alinsky in this very Freirean process, the Grandparents had achieved critical consciousnesses. The grandparents were quite confident in their quest to highlight the lack of financial help for looking after their Grandchildren and were ready to organise an event that would enable them to speak to as many people as possible including those in authority. Armitage et.al. (1999) indicates that we need to be flexible in our approach and be prepared to experiment. We have to look at the age of the group we are working with and respond accordingly.

Alinsky argued that *"...a tactic is doing what you can with what you've got."* (1971: 145) What the Grandparents had, that no one else had, was experiential stories of parenting again; this would be their weapon. To get the stories heard "*wherever possible... outside of the experience of the enemy ...*" (1971: 127) was our tactic. In practice this meant that rather than calling people to meetings where the Grandparents just moaned about their plight, something different was required, something that people would not expect and something that got everyone who attended the event involved personally.

After much discussion with the Grandparents and with all these theories and tactics in mind, 'The Story Dialogue Method' seemed bet to fit the bill perfectly as it would allow the Grandparents to remain within their experience (see Alinsky's 2nd rule on tactics, 1971:127). By telling stories well outside the experience of the invited guests and inviting reflection on them, it was hoped to catch people by surprise before they had time to switch off.

The Grandparents decided to have an event called 'Grandparents Parenting Again' to which they would invite politicians, councillors, social services and other dignitaries. The different tasks for organising this event were divided up amongst the Grandparents. We applied for and got a small grant of £1000 to help fund the venue and catering for the event. It was also decided to invite Grandparents from other councils to take part and share their experiences. The Grandparents suggested having some 'workshops' run by various agencies.

For example the Welfare Rights and the Children's Reporter ran workshops, so that visiting Grandparents and the public could valuable information and help where needed and available.

To help the Grandparents feel more comfortable telling their stories and to prepare them, we arranged a day where we went through the process of the 'Story Dialogue Method' letting the grandparents practice telling their story. This also allowed us to determine whether this method would have the impact we were hoping for and to make changes if needed.

The 'Story Dialogue Method', was refined in Canada by Labonte and Featherstone (1999). Labonte recognised that people have a wealth of expertise and experience with issues related to community development. The 'Story Dialogue method' encapsulates community development practises and values of empowerment, inclusion and social justice. It is Freirean in its approach, in that it encourages participants and audiences to progress through the three main stages of consciousness, Magical Consciousness, Naïve Consciousness and Critical Consciousness. This technique through the telling of stories, reflection and the seeking the generative theme' that really captures the issues of the community. This technique encourages people to act on that generative theme.

As people in the community, we had invited to the event, began to hear about the Grandparents a sense of excitement and willingness to help grew. Some organisations offered their services free, for example Radio Scotland offered to advertise the event for free, Midlothian Voluntary Action printed all the publicity free, the Miners Club offered their premises free. People from the community offered to hand out publicity and do door to door leafleting. The sense of ownership in the community was gratifying and seemed to vindicate the actions taken. This outcome was a strong reminder to never underestimate the power of collective action.

On the day of the Grandparents Parenting Again Event, almost every invited guest turned up, politicians of more than one political party, councillors, representatives of Scottish Executive and different agencies, grandparents from different councils and members of the public who came in to hear the debate.

Everyone was asked to sit in a large circle, making sure that the Grandparents were sitting in different places mixed in amongst the various invited guests. My colleague and I did the introductions. We explained that what we were going to do was listen to some grandparent's stories of their experience Parenting Again. Everyone was given a pen and paper to jot down notes. We wanted them to reflect on the stories given, writing down their thoughts and reactions to the stories they were hearing. The ground rules were also laid down so that the storytellers were not interrupted.

The first part of the process then was that grandparents told their stories. Stories like that of a grandparent whose estranged daughter was a heroin addict; the alarm was raised when the local G.P. couldn't get an answer at the door and the police were called as were the grandparents. The door had to be 'kicked in' and what was found was horrific, a young mother lying out cold and a three week old baby was found lying on the floor, which was covered in dog excreta, screaming. The G.P. gave the child to the grandparents who then took the child home. They stopped at a supermarket on the way home to buy baby clothes, equipment and milk, as they had nothing in the house and were not expecting to be in this situation as they did not even know they had a grandchild. Social Services arrived the next day to speak to the grandparents, when the grandparents asked for reimbursement for the baby things they had bought, they were told they were not entitled to financial help as they were family. These Grandparents only had their pension to live on and lived in a small one bedroom pensioner's house. This kind of story was not too unfamiliar to most of the people at the event.

When the grandparents had finished telling their story, we asked the audience to reflect on the stories writing down their feelings and thoughts. We then invited the grandparent from other councils to give their stories too, asking the audience to write down their reflections on those stories.

We then started the structured dialogue by asking the 'reflective' (what) questions. What were the problems and the needs of the grandparents at that time? This generated some heated discussion as politicians were asking what the local authorities were doing, then the local authorities were asking what social services were doing and so the 'buck' kept passing. The grandparents from other areas joined in the discussion saying that they had experienced the same in the 'Council Regions' they lived in.

The next part of the process was asking the 'explanation' (why) questions, like: 'why did the grandparents feel let down by social services? And: 'why were the grandparents so angry? Then more generally asking: 'why did this happen? What was interesting was how the politicians all blamed one another's economic policy on 'Kinship Care' for failing these Grandparents who were now parenting again. This was part of our strategy (using the 'Story Dialogue Method' to open up discussion.) Knowing that elections were coming up, we hoped that the politicians, at least, would see the opportunity promote their party and would want to look favourably at changing their policy on 'Kinship care' as a potential 'vote winner'.

The 'synthesis' (so what) questions came next. We asked the audience what had we learnt from the stories and the discussions and what remained confusing. What became clear was that the existing Social Policy in general was confusing, as some politicians thought the policy on financial help for foster care included Grandparent. It was becoming clear that the Local Authorities thought differently and classed Grandparents as 'family', which was very convenient as it meant they would not have to budget for any financial payments to Grandparents parenting again.

The discussion exposed that Grandparents were economic pawns in social policy debates in regard to foster care. The status quo was saving the local authorities money, as the children were living with their Grandparents without financial help, saving the Councils the foster care allowance that would be payable if the children were placed in care.

Before the discussion became too heated we moved on to 'action' (now what) questions, asking the audience: where do we go from here? How should we treat kinship care differently? Who has the power to change things? And what is the process for changing social policy? It was interesting to observe politicians from all parties promise that if they got into power they would see to make changes to social policy and enact legislation concerning kinship care as a priority.

To finish the Story Dialogue Method phase of this process and following the structured dialogue that had just taken place, we reviewed the stories and reflected on what people had written during the question time. This was to create 'insight cards' that would reflect the common themes. The importance of 'insight cards' is to enable the participants in the dialogue to see the generative theme that could propel them to action.

The Grandparents Parenting Again event closed with those who had attended taking part in the workshops enjoying a buffet together. The Grandparents were presented with the 'Group of the Year' award for Adult Learning, for organising this event.

The Story Dialogue Method worked much better than the grandparents and I could ever have imagined. While the stories were being told, it was clear from people's facial expressions that they had no idea that grandparents who were the sole carers of their grandchildren were not receiving financial help.

The telling of stories (the code) was an empowering process for the grandparents as they were able to share their experiences and encourage others to reflect on them. The 'Story Dialogue Method' can be as Labonte comments "... *powerful tool when several stories are told... around the same theme. In this way the insights generated...produce a practical action plan...*" (1999: 2). This was exactly how the Story Dialogue Method played out at the Parenting Again event. As a direct result of the insights generated by the stories, a very heated debate was provoked between the Scottish Executive's representatives, politicians and local authorities, who then started to look at practical ways to help the Grandparents.

This favourable outcome was achieved by employing the complimentary methods of Freire and Alinsky. In the quest for empowerment and conscientisation it is almost as if Alinsky draws the picture and Freire colours it in.

That was the success of using the Story Dialogue Method at the Grandparents event, because the process of leading invited guests from magical consciousness to critical consciousness, through the stories, was so unexpected, that it caught those we were trying to influence off guard. Any predetermined responses that the invited guests may have had, were rendered redundant and they were taken beyond their experience. How many events do politicians encounter where they are asked to listen to stories then asked to write their reflections on them, before a debate?

As Barr commented that community practice must be about *"...enabling and empowering community members, collectively to participate actively in response to community problems..."* (1996: 4)

The grandparents began to empower themselves through the learning circles at the beginning of the process, which prompted them to organise the Grandparents Parent Again, which in turn empowered them to challenge the existing social policy regarding financial help to grandparents parenting again.

This pluralistic perspective on empowerment fitted best our situation. As Ife explains so well this way of working means that:

> *"...everyone can have their say, all people have equal opportunity to participate, no one is all powerful... power is*

spread among...different and competing groups... empowerment is a process of helping disadvantage individuals to compete more effectively helping... to learn...skills in lobbying , ... engaging in political action." (2003: 54)

In other words *"...understanding how to work the system...".*

I would agree with Ife because the beauty of the 'Story Dialogue Method' in our case was that by the combining the ideas of Freire on empowerment through 'conscientisation' and those of Alinsky, whose work is premised on the 'pluralistic perspective' of empowerment, meant that the Grandparents took a radical approach and worked outside everyone's experience but their own.

It was suggested that the Grandparents themselves could petitioned parliament and start a debate on having changes made to social policy that would lead grandparents 'Parenting Again' being given financial help. Some of the politicians said they would help the grandparents to take this further and arrange some parliamentary training for them. They also offered to help then put together a formal report.

In the meanwhile Strathclyde and Highland councils piloted a scheme through which grandparents were given the same financial assistance as foster cares. The Fostering and Adoption policy now includes that, grandparents should be given the same rights, responsibilities and financial help as foster cares, it would be called the Kinship Care Allowance.

The Scottish National Party decided to devolve the Kinship Care Allowance funding to each of the 32 councils and allowed them to decide how the money was to be allocated. As a result some council's have not given the full allowances to all grandparents' kinship caring. This has caused frustration and a feeling of discrimination, among grandparents parenting again not receiving the full Kinship Care Allowance.

The natural progression now for the Grandparents would be to use the Elite prospective of empowerment. In regard to this perspective Ife (2003) says *"... seek alliances with powerful elites to pursue ones own ends, for example by enlisting the help of the legal profession...".* Ife also suggested that *"...politics is not a 'game' where all the players have equal opportunities to win"*. This is a very good point as at this stage the Grandparents do have not equal opportunities.

An example of how the Elite perspective of empowerment works would be in the case of two Grandparents living in England who in 2008 sought legal advice regarding taking their local council to court. Their local authority was trying to find ways of exempting the Grandparents from receiving the Kinship Care Allowance. Without this extra money the Grandparents and their Grandchildren were in real poverty. The Grandparents had tried to challenge council themselves, but were not taken seriously. By enlisting the help of the legal profession they raised the stakes.

The Grandparents won their court case and the council were told to not only pay costs but to backdate the Kinship Care Allowance to them from the date it's coming into effect. If other Grandparents were to build alliances with the legal profession and politicians and work alongside them, allowing them to challenge social policy and legislation from a legal stand point; just think how powerful that would be.

Therefore the Grandparents need to use the existing links and networks that they have across Scotland and the UK to form a constituted 'National Grandparents Group. Capitalizing on the good will of the politicians and professionals who have expressed support for the changes that need to be made in policy and legislation regarding Kinship Care, (there are some indications that, at the time of writing, this may be about to happen). By forming a National Grandparents Group it will afford them more credibility to continue lobbying parliament, encouraging changes to be made to policy and legislation concerning Kinship Care.

Note; there is now a national grandparents parenting again group that meets regularly in Glasgow, with a grandparents representative attending form each of the areas in Scotland.

Commentary

This study is important in raising the often hidden role of family in supporting the welfare system and the failings of some social policies. In doing so it provides a solid example of creative work with a social group that is if often ignored or marginalised for development activity.

The study also describes a very creative mix of theoretical process; the linking of Freire and a popular education process with a campaigning objective underpinned by the ‘rules’ of Saul Alinsky. This hybrid approach offers significant potential in turning the reflection – vision process into clear and effective action.

Practice Study 9

Chinese Community: fundraising group.

Rosemary Robertson

Abstract

This study is based on work within a Chinese community. It is focussed on supporting a small group seeking major funding for their multicultural centre.

The Study

This practice study discusses work within a Multicultural Centre. The study integrates an evaluation of practice methods within an appropriate theoretical framework. The focus of the work was to support communities to plan and take collective action and to support communities to monitor and review action for change. I shall conclude by evaluating my interventions.

The Multicultural Centre is used predominantly by the local Chinese community and focuses on social activities that integrate the community. The centre had recently signed a new lease for 10 years with the option of release after 5 years. A condition of the lease was to carry out a buildings survey to ascertain the level of repairs required and that these repairs be completed within 3 years and funded by the Hall Committee of the centre. The survey showed that £100,000 of repairs was required. The hall committee had decided to create a sub group that would support the manager in raising funds for the repairs. My role was to support the group by assisting in the creation of an action plan, which the hall committee approved.

At the initial meeting I was immediately struck by the obvious split in the group. There are five members in the group all of which are involved in the community council and three of which are members of the hall committee. Two members of the hall committee have been involved for over twenty years whilst the remaining member is a recent addition. The two other members are relatively new also. The more established members seemed cautious of the newer members and had difficulty with any ideas around processes and procedures as well as using technology for communication purposes. The newer members seemed frustrated by this as they saw modern technology as a way to advance the aims of the group. I sensed that this split could lead to future conflict and I knew that I would have to make some interventions, which could help in this area. I related the situation to Bruce Tuckman's (1965) group development model where he believes there are five stages in a group; forming, storming, performing, norming and mourning. I felt that the more established members of the group believed they were at the performing stage and wanted to go full steam ahead without necessarily planning their actions. However I felt that the group were between the forming/storming stages and that unless the group spent time communicating with each other they would not reach the performing stage.

Another issue that became apparent to me was that the group seemed to pass all decisions to the manager who would then complete any actions. This seemed to leave the manager feeling unsupported and under pressure. I was unsure as to whether this was because the group felt this was his role or that they did not feel able to take decisions for themselves or that they simply didn't think they could make their own decisions and take actions themselves. The group also had a lack of knowledge with regards to support organisations or available funding. The group had limited understanding of monitoring or review procedures. My supervisor also explained that the group might be wary of my involvement even though they had agreed to it. He advised that I tread carefully and ensure that the group understand that I was there to support the group rather than tell them what to do.

As a result of my observations I planned actions for myself which I agreed with the group and my supervisor. These were as follows:

1. Identify potential sources of support
2. Identify potential sources of funding
3. Build solid relationships based on trust with each group member
4. Assist in the development of an action plan
5. Assist in the development of a monitoring/review plan
6. Assist the group in making decisions

7. Work with the group to identify potential roles and agree how to allocate them

I also had to ensure that the work I was doing would meet the required criteria for my placement. I had initially been concerned that by trying to meet the criteria set out for me that I would be working to my own agenda rather than that of the community. However, I felt reassured once I knew that my workload was based on the needs of the group. I was comfortable that I could meet the criteria in a way that meant I was still working towards the communities' agenda.

Prior to working with the group I felt it extremely important to explore my values in relation to community work. Ledwith (2005) offers a model of critical praxis where she suggests the starting point of any practice is to explore our values and beliefs. To do this I related to the values and principle set in the Community Development National Occupational Standards (Paulo 2003). Whilst I value all of the values laid out in the standards there are a few that I relate to more. These include sustainability, participation, working and learning together and reflective practice. I feel that it is important that when working with communities we share our skills in a way that allows the community to become sustainable. It is important that when we work with groups we do not do the work for them but with them so that they can learn those skills and continue their work after my departure. I hoped that by developing a long-term action plan with the group, establishing roles and engaging with relevant support agencies, the group would indeed become sustainable. I also feel it is important that all involved have the opportunity to fully participate which means that I must identify barriers to participation and work to increase the confidence of individuals to take part. To do this I worked to build individual relationships with group members.

I hoped to create a relationship based on trust and mutual respect whereby individuals could approach me with any issues they experienced. This allowed me to identify any barriers or issues that could have prevented participation. For example, one member didn't feel she had anything to offer the group in terms of skills. I spent time talking about her experiences in community work and we discussed how she had developed excellent communication and negotiation skills as a result, which could benefit the group. This increased her confidence and she began to participate more fully in group discussions and decisions. I believe that by working and learning together we can overcome barriers such as lack of knowledge or skills as well as barriers whether they are cultural, language or other.

Lastly, I believe that to be an effective practitioner I would have to reflect on my practice on a regular basis to ensure that I am working in line with my values. I chose to do this by keeping a reflective diary that I filled in at the end of each placement day, meeting with my supervisor to discuss my practice and meeting with my placement tutor to discuss any issues and to seek guidance. This was extremely helpful as I was able to talk through my concerns and evaluate whether my interventions were effective.

The next step in the Critical Praxis model is to refer to the theorists that have influenced your practice. I have been extremely influenced by the principles of Paulo Freire as described by Hope & Timmel in Training for Transformation.

> "*Dialogue is the main way in which we develop our capacity to think and make judgements, a group is far more likely to absorb and benefit from this if the program is started with dialogue, which brings to the surface all the latent questions in their minds. A relevant input will then challenge them to deeper thinking and further dialogue*" (1995: 19).

Freire believed that dialogue around relevant issues identified by the community would lead to action. He also believed that action must be reflected upon at regular stages to ensure we meet our aims and objectives. As mentioned earlier I believed that the group were heading towards conflict due to different ideas on how to progress. I was also influenced by Rod Purcell who introduced me to the idea of Learning Circles which can be defined as:

> "*Small, on-going gatherings of people who come together to share their ideals, goals, practices and honest experiences in service learning. In all cases, learning circles seek to be free spaces where open discussion of hard questions can take place in a collaborative and enriching environment that brings together people from different constituencies*" (2005: 219) Purcell goes on to say, "*the circles provide a welcome alternative to the traditional office bearer/committee structure*

> *which tends to both dominate and restrict community groups. For participative work, learning circles can encourage user involvement through creating a supportive enabling environment*".

Purcell explains that these circles help to build people's confidence and relationships and help them to plan and take action. They are similar to the Freirean approach in that they aim to develop critical consciousness but differ from the Freirean approach in that the circles "*are less dependent upon generative themes but more focussed on immediate task and issues that need to be explored*". I felt this approach was relevant for my group. The group had already identified its issues so there was no need for a listening survey to identify generative themes or codes to feed them back. The group had identified issues they wished to take action on so it seemed that a learning circle that focussed on "*immediate tasks and issues*" was more relevant to the group. Relevance is a critical factor for Freire and I too believe that it leads to action because, like with this group, it creates passion and motivation.

To encourage dialogue through a learning circle environment I arranged sessions where the group had the opportunity to share their issues, values and hopes. This was done out with formal group meetings and therefore free of the restrictions of office bearers, minute taking and formal processes. I posed questions for the group in speed dating exercises where each person had the opportunity to talk to every member of the group. This was successful in that the group found common values and shared beliefs. It was a way to overcome barriers to participation, as each person was able to discuss their concerns and receive reassurance from each other. I observed the group bonding with one another and my previous concerns about potential conflict were eased now that the group seemed to value one another and their contributions.

The group expressed through evaluations at the end of each session that they found the learning circles extremely valuable in terms of creating understanding of each other and bonding as a group. However, they still felt it important that they function in a more traditional way when it came to actual meeting around the action group. They agreed to keep the learning circles as a regular session to develop the group but that they would use the formal approach to develop their action plan and meet their objectives.

The main aim of the group was to raise funds for hall repairs. The group lacked knowledge of funding sources or organisations that could offer support in this area. They had relied on one source of funding from the City Council for almost 20 years and this funding had been subject to regular cuts from an annual budget of £70,000 to just £50,000. I realised that the group may need to address other funding issues as well as the funding required for the repairs. I researched support organisations and found the local office of the Community Planning Partnership (CPP) as well as local Regeneration Agency (GWRA).

I provided the group with information on these organisations and they agreed to make contact and arrange meetings. I found out which councillor sat on the funding executive group for CPP and we invited him to a meeting to ask him to offer information and support to the group, he has now become a regular attendee at the meetings and has begun a process of discussions with the group.

A meeting was arranged with an advisor from GWRA who gained an initial overview of the organisation. She advised that the group carry out an Organisational Health Check and that on completion of this, they would make recommendations towards a long-term action plan. The group had limited or in some cases no experience of action planning. In the learning circle we had clarified the aims and objectives of the group and we used this to create an initial action plan. During this session I encouraged everyone to participate by asking the group to develop a mind map that could be used to develop an action plan. I also used a participatory appraisal method, which was a talking wall. I used flipcharts with specific questions and the group were put in teams and asked to write their answers on the flipcharts. This too was used to develop the action plan. It was effective in that the informality encouraged the group to participate. It also got the group working in teams where they had to discuss their answers and agree to them before they were added.

The group agreed that we develop and use this short-term action plan until the Health Check was complete and we had received recommendations from GWRA along with their initial ideas on the support that they could provide. The initial action plan included aims to create an online email group, information letters explaining the situation to several audiences, raising awareness of the issue, gathering support from relevant politicians, a group agreement, and detailed who would carry out each task and the timeline for each task.

This was effective in helping the group to use an action plan process without it being too large a task. It was also a good way to introduce the group to monitoring processes as we had clear goals and outcomes that could be monitored. All of this would be great experience for the development of the long-term action plan and help the group to recognise that using processes can be an advantage to them. I believe that by using the learning circle method the group were able to move from a forming stage to a performing stage where they were able to see progress and use the information gathered in the learning circles to develop their action plan. I introduced the group to the concept of reviewing and monitoring by asking the group to begin each group with a review of the previous meeting and progress made since. I asked them to carry out an evaluation at the end of each meeting where they would look at the effectiveness of their decision-making and performance as a group.

The group participated well in this and it was a gentle way to begin the process of encouraging them to think about monitoring. I then asked the group to participate in a session on monitoring which I would facilitate. I asked the group to consider the purpose of monitoring. I didn't want to assume that the group had no experience of this therefore I asked if they had and one member had extensive experience through his job. He shared this with the group who were then able to ask questions and relate those experiences to the groups monitoring requirements.

I introduced the group to S.M.A.R.T (Haughey 2009) which is a process which helps create, specific, measurable, achievable, realistic and timed goals which can set the criteria for monitoring. This is a simple process and the group agreed that this was a method they would use when developing their long-term action plan.

The group began to create a monitoring plan. This included regular reviews of the action plan, regular evaluation sessions and a logbook to record actions between meetings. A later session saw the group agree on methods of how to feedback this information to the community and it was agreed that minutes would be put on the Community Council website, one member of the group would feed back to the Management Committee and that the group would attend community events to publicise the groups progress.

Initially I had been concerned that the group would resent being asked to monitor their progress, as it is an alien concept to the majority of them. However I was pleasantly surprised by their positive response, which taught me that I should be careful not to make judgement about a group as this may prevent me from trying out different methods with future groups. The evaluation carried out at the end of the session provided me with extremely positive feedback. One participant explained that she felt the session was a "*real learning curve*" and she had enjoyed this type of meeting, which was unlike any she'd been to before.

The group explained that they were comfortable with the agreed monitoring plan but that this too should be subject to review to ensure its effectiveness along the line. This session also saw the group exploring the potential roles that could be required in the group, what these roles would consist of and how they would be allocated. The group spent time exploring this but agreed that they required more time to think about this and would come together at another meeting to discuss it further. I wondered if this was because they liked the style of the learning circles however they later explained that they did feel they required specific roles to be allocated but that it would be better to wait until the long-term action plan had been developed to ensure that everyone had a clear understanding of the requirements of each role.

The organisational health check is now complete and the group awaits recommendations from GWRA. Work has been completed on a funding application, which can be used as a template for others. I have supported the group with this as well as identifying further funding sources. I have helped the group access long-term support, which will help them become sustainable after my departure. Overall I feel that my interventions have been valuable in that the group now have processes in place and feel optimistic about their ability to meet their aims. They are working more effectively as a group and I feel confident that they will continue to do so. In relation to my values and the values of community development the group have become more sustainable, are working and learning together as I had hoped and are participating in an inclusive manner.

In retrospect I feel that the group has made excellent progress. I was able to build their confidence in their abilities whilst encouraging them to build useful processes into their practice. I have every confidence that the group will succeed and have even agreed to support them in developing their long-term action plan once my involvement had ended. By working with communities we encourage participation, working and learning together, social justice, sustainability, pride, love and ultimately positive change. I am proud to have learned this and it certainly impacted on my practice:

> "*Every living person has some gift or capacity of value to others. A strong community is a place that recognises these gifts and ensures they are given. A weak community is a place where lots of people can't or don't give their gifts."*
>
> *"Every single person has capacities, abilities and gifts. Living a good life depends on whether those capacities can be used, abilities expressed and gifts given"*(McKnight and Kretzmann).

Commentary

This study is very clear that effective practice is based on the application of core community development values. In addition, good practice needs to be informed by the critical use of theory (critical praxis).

There were a number of group work challenges embedded in this work and the process for understanding the issues, planning responses and sensitively taking action are explored in detail.

The study also raises important questions on the value of short term and clearly focussed interventions, and the need for clarity on the distribution of role between worker(s) and community members.

Practice Study 10

East Ayrshire Council's Community Learning and Development team focusing on community capacity building

Lisa Peet

Abstract

This study is based within a local authority CLD team with the focus on capacity building within, and between, local community associations.

The Study

This practice study is based within East Ayrshire Council's Community Learning and Development team focusing on community capacity building. The team consisted of five community development workers, who were responsible to a senior worker and a manager, who in turn managed other staff; youth workers, a Gaelic tutor, and street youth workers.

The Community Development team (CLAD) is an all encompassing generic team and have three strands that they work with:

1. Adult learners.
2. Youth Work.
3. Community Capacity building.

There were two focuses of this work:

1. Facilitate a forum for the FAM support group and action outcomes.
2. To work with two community associations towards collective action on a national initiative - Adult Learners Week.

Initially, I was invited to sit in on a meeting with my manager to gain an understanding the WALT; the working and learning together guidance for community development that also supports adult literacy and numeracy (Scottish Executive 2004).

All work in the department is delivered to the local community is underpinned by the National Occupational Standards for Community Development Work (Paulo 2003). This is incorporated with work plans, and individual action plans, that are support by HGIOCLAD and LEAP frameworks.

LEAP (Learning Evaluation and Planning) is participatory and needs led tool that enables workers and communities to plan, evaluate and reflect in a continuous cycle to action outcomes, this is a framework that responds to the HMIE report: Adult literacy and numeracy in Scotland 2005 (LEAP.2006: 8). The HGIOCLAD is a self evaluation framework as a means of assessing the impact of the work (service delivery) and how I would implement it, by using the indicators to assess strengths and weaknesses of the proposed work. This document is open to internal inspection of the HMIE and copies are given to the manager. This is supported internally with individual action plans and regular team manager's report. (Scottish Government 2006).

The first aim was to facilitate a forum for the FAM (a family carer action group) for parents whose children have learning disabilities. It had been identified that there was a need to re-evaluate the groups aim and objectives due to member's ongoing concerns about the direction of the group and lack of focus.

The forum day was my first meeting with the group and initially the group were quiet but using active listening and icebreakers that I had used previously in my youth work setting I was able to make the group feel comfortable and relaxed. I feel this was shown through their steady and increased participation through the morning.

After a productive session, three areas for development were identified by the group:

- Publicity drive
- Advocacy and support for families
- Future roles and way forward for FAM

We arranged another meeting at a convenient day and time with group members; this was to look into the publicity drive. The group felt that the key to the survival of the group would rest on the capacity to build up the membership, with the hope that new members would take on office bearer's roles. By the end of the meeting the group appeared empowered and this was reflected in the evaluation.

The session was productive although I didn't want to be giving the group any false hopes in that the issues highlighted were resolved as they were not. Therefore in the planning and implementation stage of the forthcoming session, I spent time pre-empting the possible outcomes and how we could best deal with these.

I spent time doing three separate session plans based on the outcomes of the forum, and hoped that by making people feel valued it could raise their self esteem. In turn would have a positive effect on the group in terms of participation. This entailed using clear session plans to divide the facilitating between me and my supervisor, so I could also have the opportunity to listen and feedback to the group on my observations.

Discussing the session plan in detail with my supervisor, it became ever more apparent that this meeting would be the pinnacle to the development or folding of this group. I had spent three days working on the session plans and felt really happy with myself that I had put in this much preparation, as I wanted the meeting to be positive and constructive for the group.

The meeting day arrived and only two members turned up, (one dropped in for a coffee) this wasn't enough of a representation to go forward. So the chairperson and I had a meeting to discuss thoughts of the day and the session plan. The chair agreed to send letters to each member to ensure they knew the future date of the proposed meeting, and could forward plan for it.

Later I was advised by my supervisor and the chair, after phone calls to members it was highly unlikely that any more than two members would attend a further meeting, so therefore it was not worth going ahead, as it is not possible to sustain a group with 2 members and a chair person.

I initially felt sad that this had happened, but the member's non-intention of turning up the meetings, in retrospect answered the question regarding the probability of the group folding. I spent time speaking in supervision about the cycle of groups and how the folding of the group was realistic and appropriate at that time, as it had done what it had originally set out to do and this was its natural ending. I was able to have an exit meeting with the chair who also voiced the same issue about groups that my supervisor did and felt it was expected.

I used the learning loop to look at the cycle of the group and using this I conclude it had gone 'full circle', so if the group continued it would need to re-establish the visions, values and goals and once in the reflection. I could see that it had met its original aim of being a campaigning organisation. It had enabled the 'birth and growth' of a group run by and for the children and adults with learning disabilities (VIP). So the closure of this group enabled the path for VIP group.

In reflection I feel now that the forum day should of really been based around 'evaluate the effect of the group in relation to the VIP group', and then perhaps they would have agreed to fold and done that in a fun or social event way, rather than dissolving with no proper ending, which I didn't feel was constructive for the group or individuals.

This was the first time I had ever been involved in a group that had folded and I feel the experience has been very useful for my further understanding of how to accept the cycle of groups.

The second focus was to work with two local community associations and support them to work collectively to facilitate a joint open day for the forthcoming Adult Learners Week (ALW) to be held in local community centre.

At this time there was a new service level agreement drawn up by the council and I was able to have a meeting with one of the service managers to explain the reasons for the service level agreements. I found this valuable and helpful, as I had not previously worked with community associations and it was a new experience, and an opportunity to gain an insight into the history of associations in Ayrshire.

Alan Twelvetrees has commented that:

> *"In Scotland there appears to be a strong historical link to education and community centres. Community associations have come through the ages since; Edinburgh's education department provided temporary centres in the early 1950's, but the association were only allowed to use the centres under certain conditions".* (1976: 33)

This has moved with the times as now the community associations have a constitution and service level agreement in which explains their terms and conditions of office. Although drawn up by the council they need to discuss and agree these documents. I feel this gives the members a degree of power from their perspective. Although looking at this using Arnstein's ladder of participation I feel that it is a degree of tokenism, rather than a degree of citizenship power, as the consultation stage was one meeting and now each member was advised to read and sign the document (Dailly 1992). The consequence for not signing the document means that the council would withdraw services, i.e. community development worker, caretakers and maintaining the building. Therefore they don't really have a choice, as they couldn't manage the centre without support.

The associations (CA1 and CA2) are two neighbouring villages that are geographically one mile apart. Before meeting with them, I met with my supervisor who gave me a brief overview of the association as she wanted me to feedback to her my thoughts and feeling of the groups and what I see happening. My supervisor had already spoken to the groups prior to my start to ask if they would be willing to speak with me about proposed work and both were willing to do this.

I met all the members of CA1 (apart from the chair who was ill) and CA2, by attending both of the community association regular meetings and AGM's. I also helped out on a psychic night with CA2 and organised a litter pick as part of the national 'keep Scotland tidy campaign' with CA1. This I felt was a good way for me to give something back to the associations, to show that I was interested in what they do and willing to help as much as much as the members, this also gave them time to get to know me as well.

This was a good opportunity to see how each of the groups worked and who the dominant members of the groups were, as I was aware from meeting's that there was a silent minority, I used Tuckman's (1965) model of group work to help me understand the dynamics of the group. Tuckman describes groups as working in five stages, but I felt after observing both associations that CA1 was at the storming stage as they could not agree democratically on a decision, and CA2 were at the performing stage as they were willing to work together and were already thinking of events to plan for the following year.

Through discussions there appeared to be resistance from CA1 towards working together, so I decided I needed to find out why and I would need to try and continue to build relationship and acceptance for people to feel confident and explain the issues of CA1 towards CA2.

The majority of members form CA1 was also not happy with the venue being pre-arranged to be held at CA2 centre, and this had been published on poster information without consultation; considering one of the values of community development was about participation and respect I felt disappointed that this had happened.

This gave my supervisor an opportunity to explain why there had been no consultation with the groups and it was a matter of practicality, as CA1 had bingo and chair aerobic on the Wednesday so would not cancel them and the other centre was not in use. She did accept that this was a learning point for the team as they had chosen the day and place and in retrospect they should not have done this, and it was agreed I would feed this back to the association members at the next scheduled meetings.

I spent much time speaking one to one with the members of CA1 in an aim to understand the feelings of resistance towards workingg with CA2, and to see if there would be a way forward in terms of collective action and working between the two associations. As Hope and Timmel comment *"participants' in groups need the courage to speak up when that have had little participation in the form of democracy"* (1995: 123).

It transpired during the phone calls that the 'group' reason for not wanting to be part of anything to do with the other association, was down to a long standing dispute about CA2 not supporting an environmental group that CA1 were very passionate about starting.

A lot of work went into promoting and organising the environmental day event but on the day not one person turned up from the public or the other association. This lack of support appears to have driven a wedge between collective working and action. As members of CA1 had been left feeling undervalued, dejected and embarrassed. A more vocal member of CA1 was adamant that "*it (ALW) wouldn't work, so there was no point, as local people would not attend, and the other association wouldn't help either, so no point having it in our centre*"(committee member). Twelvetrees states that *"emotionally over involved people are to a large degree meeting their own needs, when issues arise they take it personally and blame the people for whose benefit it should benefit"* (2002: 63).

I felt that it would be useful to invite each group to their own association's meeting, to see if we could move on from this pit-stop and see if collaborative working could be achieved. Or if not decide on the next strategy to enable them to feel valued, as the work they do is appreciated, regardless of if they would work together.

This meeting went ahead with CA1 and five members out of a possible 12 turned up, to which I was quite surprised and a little disappointed, as previously on the phone members had clarified turn out, after explaining the idea for collective working.

At the meeting, I had the opportunity to discuss ALW in detail and the roles available for them to take on, if they wished. I decided to prepare a 'list' of jobs to do for the event this would be a good way of getting people talking and seeing who would be more comfortable in different roles, also it takes the pressure off the day as everyone will be clear about what their role was. All members were quite willing to meet up with CA2 next week to implement the details of a plan for ALW.

Two members who I had previously spoken to, on the phone were not in attendance as they were at work and the practicalities of attending ALW was impossible for them, so they took on the role of designing leaflet and volunteering to do the 'leaflet drop'. Two other members would be on holiday; therefore they did not see the point in being part of the sub group.

When I met with the members of CA2 they were different altogether and had not realised there were feelings of animosity, so I decided not to tell them as I didn't feel it would be constructive to their learning, and the members from CA1 that were wanting to be part of joint working exercise were not of the same opinion as their peers. All members from CA2 wanted to participate; they were open and looking forward to working together.

The joint meeting went ahead and was a positive experience from the verbal feedback by all Members. It was constructive and in one session they were able to decide the roles for the event day and what they would like to put on display boards, who was serving tea/coffee, some decided to drop leaflets and others decided who to invite (groups) to have a stall and be part of it, they even arranged for a 'taster Reiki' session for people who attended.

At a further meeting the group were also able to decide on how to evaluate the event and how they felt the public would best respond. They decided to ask people to write comments on post it notes, as they didn't feel this was too time consuming, this would also give them something to discuss at the evaluation session after the event. The event went ahead successfully and out of the small numbers of attendees, all signed up to make a commitment to adult learning.

My role as an educator entailed me to be open and engaging with the group, not just a listener who sits on the fence, but having the ability to think about the context of what people are saying and challenging assumption, which clearly I needed to do in a positive manner otherwise the sub group would not have formed. This is why I made an informed decision to phone people and speak to them as individuals. (Jeffs & Smith 1999).

To make changes we all need to be open to new things, I felt I supported and encouraged them to the best of their ability and I used a reflective journal and supervision session with my supervisor to question my thoughts and actions.

Throughout my practice I used the Johari Window model (by Ingham and Luft) to assess how I was feeling and what could people see about me and in particular my blind self (Daily 1992). As I had an expectation of the group members to be open and honest about what they expected from the event, therefore I was conscious of what my role, and my reasons for wanting the collective action to go ahead, what I needed to question was my integrity to do it so it was constructive for both of the associations and its members.

My hope was that this piece of work impacted positively and enables the groups to feel valued and encourage them to identify other needs for their community and further collective action. I was able to feed back to the group the positive learning outcomes of the event using a clear session plan and allowing time for people to speak.

I decided I would use Kolb's (1984) experiential learning cycle to assess the process of collective action and the impact on the group. Kolb defines learning as *"the process whereby knowledge is created through the transformation of experience*" (Tight 1996: 99). Kolb's cycle has four stages, but my starting point was 'observing and reflecting' (point 2), as I was assessing the dynamics of the group and how they worked, moving on the theories of their behaviours i.e. hostility towards CA2, and by using transferable skills from other roles I have undertaken I was able to listen, engage and enable the individuals to explore and move on to 'test new situations', the collective action and the experience.

This leads to the reflection stage and I can now compare the autonomy of the group to assess if this experience had a positive impact, using the evaluation session. Hope & Timmel suggest that "*evaluation should be as supportive and not destructive*". Therefore I was very conscious when organising the evaluation session and deciding on which method to use to feedback the information.

I decided that 'dialogical evaluation' (Jeffs & Smith) I felt this was the most appropriate method, as the group was autonomous adult individuals, working for a common goal, and having been through the process it would be useful for us as educators and participants to hear our views on this experiences of this journey. It enabled everyone to explore their feelings about the experience and what conclusion they have come to.

The group as a whole thought the experience was positive and ended their evaluation session by planning for future collective work; they started to explore other initiatives and events that they could hold the following year, as it would be more beneficial to their local communities in respect of what they would want. I also think this enables people to feel valued, as during many of the meetings evaluations were discussed and issues about 'evaluation just being a paper exercise', therefore this wouldn't work for this groups, they needed closure to this piece of work to enable them to look forward to the future.

I feel that some of the members had not been active within their associations before the collective action and therefore didn't really understand the democratic process, rather followed the more dominant members in the group. Therefore this reflection on action process, where they are now able to look back at work and asses it before deciding the next step has and will continue to have an impact on their learning and future ventures.(Hope & Timmel).

I agree with the following statement: "*A community centre can be considered a focal point of the community or the 'heart' of it",* (Twelve trees. 1976: 21) *but the passion comes from the people who run it.* In relation to the Community development principles, I feel that the community associations demonstrated their commitment to collective working under the following headings:

Participation

I felt I enabled participation and took time to ensure this was highlight in the session plans. By choosing to be an active part of Adult learner's week and advertising the good work that the associations do to encourage the uptake of the local activities and classes and support people to ask for new classes. All ages and abilities were invited to the event from across both the villages and members actively designed and posted leaflets.

Working and learning together

Both of the associations undertook a huge piece of work in their already busy schedules to promote the event, they overcame barriers to working together and enabled learning from each other, with the hope it will be done again in the future but at a central location in the town as they felt this would encourage a larger turnout, as easier to get to on the bus.

Sustainable communities

Both associations' members in the sub group promoted effective collective and collaborative working by using themselves as an example of what can be achieved, this also became part of the evaluation session for members to be reflective and learn from their experience and make changes for the future.

Reflective practice

By attending the final session in which the evaluation of the whole experience took place all members were able to assess what they would do differently next time. I feel this was a crucial piece of work for me as the facilitator to enable them to leave the experience feeling valued and empowered for future causes.

Self determination

I feel that I valued the members concerns and issues that they had in respect of working collectively and feel this was handled in a sensitive nature and allowed positive outcomes' for the groups.

I feel that with my support the associations members were empowered to show a commitment to raising people's awareness of choices open to them was extremely encouraging as a worker and they were able to discuss the 'bigger picture' in respect of continuing education and what they felt the local people wanted. Then main item was how they could do this again using another location, although it did urge them to look into putting a similar event on in relation to:

Social justice

I feel that the I encouraged the members to take into account all ability is of their local communities and respecting the limits of what people can do, by offering opportunities for designing leaflets and delivering them, as I was mindful some peoples fitness abilities were not similar but being supportive so I gave a list to members in which streets I would deliver to and what they wanted to do, being speakers on the event day and enabling an evaluation opportunity to assess what did happen and learn from it.

I thought the process of me being a catalyst to support both associations worked well and I feel this was due to the time I depend building relationships with themselves and valuing their thoughts and feelings, using the models of group work and support from my supervisor.

Commentary

As would be expected from local authority based work, the approach is well structured, planned and with inbuilt approaches to evaluation. The study is very honest in confronting the difficulties of involving group members and general members of the public in activities that are not directly related to local issues. Adult Learning Week is a good thing, but not necessarily important to people who live locally.

The study also draws out the potential for work that has a tight local focus of hostility / competition between groups who may see themselves in competition. Of particular note is the flexible and thoughtful approach to evaluation.

Practice Study 11

Community Voices Training Programme

Iain Cunningham and Davina Hepson

Abstract

This practice study explores the work of a Community Action Team whose role is to support the development and sustainability of local community organisations. In particular the study looks at the training element of the team's activity and its impact on community groups and volunteers.

The study is written in a very formal way. As such it reflects, and provides an excellent insight into, the operational nature of the organisation and the style of work currently generated through many of the Community Planning Partnerships in Scotland.

The Study

Introduction

Section 1 of this report explains the Background of the training programme in relation to national policy.

Section 2 of this report discusses PPRC as an organisation, and its role within the Community Planning Processes.

Section 3 of this report details the role of the Community Action Team and its' function within PPRC and their linkages to community groups and Community Planning Processes.

Section 4 of this report looks at how CAT operating plan objectives are monitored and assessed.

Section 5 of this report highlights the 'Broad Principles' of the Community Voices programme and the 'National Standards of

Community Engagement' reflected within the Community Voices Programme.

Section 6 of this report describes the Community Voices training programme in practice and the Community Action Team's support to the development and sustainability of community groups and volunteers.

Section 7 of this report will examine the Community Voices programmes analysis tools and their effectiveness in identifying and removing barriers to learning through the use of case studies.

Strategic fit Background

Scottish Executive Renfrewshire Community Planning Partnership Regeneration Outcome Agreement (ROA) 2005-2008 (mission)

In August 2004 Communities Scotland issued detailed guidance on producing a three-year Regeneration Outcome Agreement (ROA) by Community Planning Partnerships. The purpose of the ROA was to set out a strategic and operational framework for the delivery of the Scottish Executive's "Closing the Opportunity Gap" document objective of:-

> **(Vision)**
> ***Regenerating the most disadvantaged neighbourhoods, so that people living there can take advantage of job opportunities and improve their quality of life.***
> (Source:
http://www.scotland.gov.uk/Publications/2002/06/14990/8017)

Single Outcome Agreement (SOA) 2008-2011

The SOA between the Scottish Government and Renfrewshire Council sets out priorities which focus on the delivery of better outcomes for the people in Renfrewshire. The purpose of the SOA is to set out a strategic and operational framework for the delivery of Scottish Governments' Concordat with the Convention of Scottish Local Authorities (COSLA) Source: Renfrewshire's Single Outcome Agreement (2008 – 2011)

Governance of the SOA for Renfrewshire is the responsibility of Renfrewshire Council. Renfrewshire Community Plan Leadership group also have a role on governance arrangements within the context of the Community Plan. (2008 – 2017)

Public service agencies contribute to of the governance SOA through their senior management teams by monitoring their contributions towards achieving the fifteen national outcomes.
Source: Renfrewshire single outcome agreement (2008 – 2011)

About PPRC

Located in Ferguslie Park in the north of Paisley (PPRC) is a registered charitable company limited by Guarantee. The company's previous focus was on area based Community Planning issues. Service was delivered thematically within 11 geographical areas of deprivation in accordance with the Scottish Index of Multiple Deprivation 2004 (SIMD ref/bib 1) 5%-15% data zones in Renfrewshire. Service Delivery was also in accordance with the then 'Scottish Executive's' 'closing the opportunity gap' document, and funded through the Community Regeneration Fund (CRF) focusing on one or more of the following national priorities, as appropriate to local circumstances and priorities:

- Building strong, safe and attractive communities;
- Getting people back into work;
- Improving health
- Raising educational attainment
- Engaging young people, for example through arts, sport and physical activity

In April 2008 the area of delivery was expanded to include Renfrewshire as a whole with 'accelerated impact' of service delivery aimed at the most disadvantaged. This process ensures that PPRC is in line with the new Scottish Government's Concordat and Renfrewshire Council's SOA guidelines and Community Plan.

PPRC provides support to Renfrewshire's Community Planning Partnership (RCPP) in its task of regenerating the most disadvantaged areas of Renfrewshire. PPRC also assists in the distribution of the Scottish Governments 'Fairer Scotland Fund' allocation for Renfrewshire. These funds are distributed to projects & initiatives that meet with the CPP's aim of promoting social inclusion in Renfrewshire's most disadvantaged areas.

Toward the end of the 1990s the concept of social exclusion became part of the UK policy context. Under the influence of the French, the term emerged out of the European Anti-Poverty Programme during the late 1980s. The French use of 'social exclusion' originates within its social policy which emphasises the need for people to have strong ties with their family and culture. Later it became associated with more structural factors concerned with the marginalisation of particular groups in urban areas. Henderson and Thomas (2003: 8).

The preceding Scottish Executive, now the Scottish Government promotes the use of the term 'promoting social inclusion' rather than that of 'tackling social exclusion', basically because the former is more upbeat. The Scottish Government's Key Priorities for communities contained within the SOA are:

- Safer and Stronger
- Wealthier and Fairer
- Healthier
- Greener
- Smarter

PPRC as a supporting and service delivery organisation has entered into a Service Level Agreement (SLA) with the Local Authority, "The Company" objectives and associated SLA targets are in line with the Government's three priorities for tackling poverty and deprivation.

- **Regenerating deprived communities**
  To support the RCPP structures that relate to regeneration, community development and employment

- **Improving employability**
  To provide support and development to local community groups to enable them to build capacity and deliver services at a local level, to assist individuals access and sustain employment and support work-force plus programmes

- **Improving life chances**
  Develop a project portfolio and co-ordinate partner activity in line with the SOA

CAT Fairer Scotland Fund

The finalised SOA details how the Fairer Scotland Fund will be utilised in Renfrewshire in conjunction with mainstream budgets & services of Community Planning Partners to regenerate Renfrewshire as a whole and have an 'accelerated impact' service delivery to the most disadvantaged.

PPRC's CAT is now 100% funded by the Fairer Scotland Fund (FSF).

The FSF brings together seven previous funding streams, these were:

Community regeneration fund
Community Voices work force plus
Changing children's service fund
Financial inclusion
More choices more chances
Working for families

The CAT is charged with engagement, capacity building and service delivery to Renfrewshire's community groups including the previous administrations Community Voices (CV) training programme element.

The predecessor to the CV fund was the Community Empowerment Fund (CEF) designed to strengthen community participation in Social Inclusion Partnerships (SIPs). In particular it sought to ensure that community representatives could play a full and equal part in partnerships. It was used in a variety of ways to provide practical support to community representatives. The fund provided £60k to each of the SIPs from 2001/02 to 2003/04. A one year extension was given during 2004/05 enabling an evaluation of community engagement in SIP's to be carried out.

The evaluation reported that:

• No one size fits all and community engagement practice will vary according to the context and community

• There is a need to provide on going support to sustain community engagement, including the investment of time and resources

•The CEF was a valuable resource to engage local people in SIPs, both by communities and agencies

•There is a need to record outcomes to demonstrate that community involvement is making a difference and influencing decisions.

•There needs to be a planned and co-coordinated approach to engaging with communities in community engagement

The new CV programme takes account of the findings of the evaluation and builds on the success of the CEF. (Source:http://www.communitiesscotland.gov.uk/stellent/groups/public/documents/webpages/otcs_012021.pdf)

The CV training programme became part of CAT activity as part of the Local Authority's duty to consult and cooperate with public bodies and community groups. The evaluation of the CEF emphasized the need to plan and coordinate activities.

In February 2005, Malcolm Chisholm, Minister for Communities 2004 – 2007 approved a new three year fund to help people living in the most disadvantaged communities to influence and engage in the planning and delivery of services and other regeneration activity in their neighbourhoods. Funding was allocated to Community Planning Partnerships.

The CV programme is operated by the CAT to support the delivery of the ROA.
The CV fund is contained within the FSF.

Performance assessment & objectives links

The CAT is a strategic operating Unit within PPRC. Performance assessment is based on a yearly objectives operating plan, this is monitored quarterly. Objectives are set & agreed by CAT staff, CAT line-manager and Renfrewshire Council's external supervising officer.

At the end of each quarter the extent to which the CAT's objectives have been met is assessed. Overall performance is based on the team's rather than individual team member's targets. Pre-set, targets are needs led in consultation with the community. This means that one officer could be delivering more of these targets than another depending on the needs of the community.

CAT targets are linked to the SOA/CPP strategies both of which are linked to Scottish Governments' FSF documents. SOA/CPP strategies are designed to provide a strategic framework that links the national priorities for tackling disadvantage, with spend and activities through the FSF and partner mainstream resources aimed at improving outcomes for disadvantaged areas and groups.

PPRC – CAT Objectives are:

- 5 Key priorities
- Support/ facilitate partnership structures
- Support/monitor projects funded by FSF
- Develop new projects
- Attract external funding

- Work with community groups
- Accelerated Impact re-Scottish Index for Multiple Deprivation 5 – 15 % target areas (SIMD)

All of the above link strategic regeneration objectives between the SOA/CPP, FSF and the 5 national priorities for regeneration all of the above link into the SIMD target areas.

The flow chart below shows how objectives are linked & communications are disseminated from Scottish Government down & from Communities up

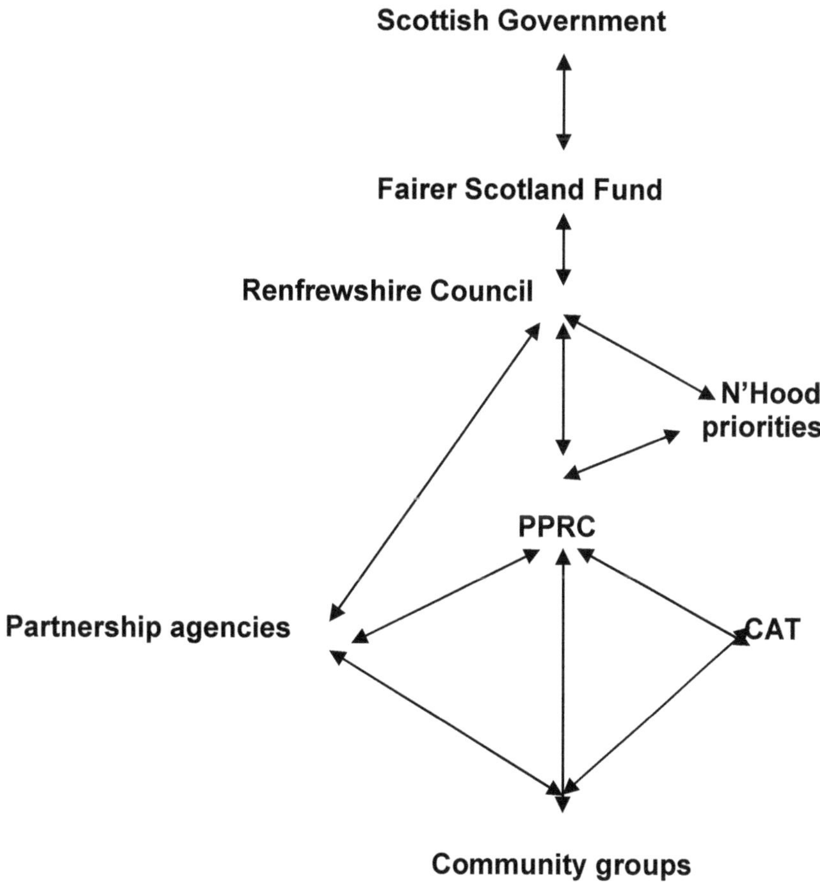

The Broad Principles of the CV Programme

Activities should be properly planned to ensure that local people have a genuine influence over the regeneration of their communities; It should provide additional support to complement existing partner support and activities related to community engagement; the National Standards for Community Engagement and related materials.

Community representatives are invaluable in their local communities, activities the programme can support include: *Training and personal / group development*: This could be informal and or formal training, for example study visits to other partnerships, undertaking accredited / non accredited or relevant training, enabling peer supporting and mentoring etc. (Source: Communities Scotland ref/bib 2)

The National Standards for Community Engagement

The principles of the National Standards for Community Engagement have been summarised as:

> *Principles that highlight the importance of equality, recognising the diversity of people and communities; a clear sense of purpose; effective methods for achieving change; building on the skills and knowledge of all those involved; commitment to learning for continuous improvement.*
> Source: National Standards for Community Engagement

The way in which the CV training programme reflects the principles of the national standards for community engagement will be evident throughout this report.

Community Voices Training in Practice

CV training was piloted in January – March 2006. After the pilot period a need for traditional training courses was identified through the use of training needs surveys of local community groups. Community groups in Renfrewshire were originally targeted and offered training such as

Committee Skills, Confidence Building, food hygiene, book keeping and literacy support and basic IT. The CAT has supported community groups in regeneration outcome areas since 1998.

Prior to 2005 data zone areas were known a Social Inclusion Partnership Areas (SIP's) Throughout 2004 area based regeneration funding was transferred from SIP's to CPPs. Support to group development i.e. drawing up a constitution, bookkeeping, applying for funding and how the community planning process works, is carried out by area based CAT Officers. This support helps community groups to sustain and build the group's capacity. Group representatives are supported to become involved in the community. CAT Officers work with groups helping them to understand of what the Community Planning process involves and how affects their communities.

The CV programme officially started on the 1st of April 2006. All groups and active volunteers residing in the 5% - 15% data zone areas in Renfrewshire were now being targeted by the CAT. Volunteers were included because it was identified that people who volunteer their time for various groups may not necessarily be group members however they are people who help run community groups. Examples of volunteers in the community are: youth workers, support workers and event organisers.

Potential CV participants are informed through their CAT Officer via word of mouth, email, PPRC e-bulletins, leaflets and information sessions. Other agencies i.e. Community Learning and Development, Community Health Partnerships, volunteer agencies, various community organisations and PPRC's Equal Access to Employment Team are also informed of training opportunities.

ll of these groups, agencies and organisations can contact the CAT and arrange a Training Needs Analysis (TNA) meeting for their clients.

The purpose of the CV training programme is to engage groups and volunteers in Renfrewshire in training and education they request during their TNA meeting. The training is not prescribed by the CAT however it should be stated that participants are asked to take part in training identified by them that will help sustain their group and build on the group's capacity. Courses are organised for group members and volunteers by the CAT. Participants can choose courses from the most commonly requested courses on the TNA or they can participate in the development of new courses that meet their group's specific needs.

The Training Needs Analysis

Initially the TNA listed only the type of training opportunities that were traditionally organised by CAT Officers. The TNA changes frequently to take account of identified needs of the community. Participants are asked to state the type of training that would benefit them and their group and why. CV participants name the training or education in a box on the TNA marked [other course] this encourages participants to state the learning they want to undertake as the TNA form cannot cover all learning experiences. This [other] box on the TNA is very useful to the CAT, through discussion each group or volunteer is encouraged to be assertive and give details of what type of training they think will benefit them and the group.
Brazilian Educator Paulo Freire refers to a cycle of action-reflection-action 'Praxis' and believes this cycle to be central to liberatory education. One characteristic of praxis is self-determination as opposed to coercion.

The TNA questions the participant's reasons for involvement i.e. *why do you think that the course you have chosen will help to benefit you or your group?*

Below are six randomly chosen sample answers to the above question:

> 1. I volunteer at a community gym and I am very interested in learning about how to deal with sports injuries.
> 2. The group needs a first aider in case one of the children gets injured I also want to learn about youth work because I volunteer in a youth club.
> 3. I want to learn to work better as part of a team and I chose mental health first aid because I think that every volunteer should be aware of mental health issues.
> 4. It can be difficult to find training as a volunteer youth worker so this is ideal.
> 5. To meet new people, build on my confidence and social skills and get more ideas about the group getting more involved in the community.
> 6. I need a food hygiene certificate to enable the nursery to run a café at fetes.

TNA questions are also intended to promote praxis while group members and the CAT Officer engage in dialogue. Discussion not only centres on the group's chosen course/s and how undertaking the course/s will benefit them when involved in their group work activity but also addresses the many barriers to learning encountered by individual participants. Barriers to learning will be discussed in more detail later.

The CAT Officer works with CV participants and tutors resulting in the type of training courses changing or developing in response to identified needs of CV participants.

According to Freire:

"In the 'Banking' concept of education, knowledge is
a gift by those who consider themselves knowledgeable
upon those whom they consider to know nothing.
Projecting an absolute ignorance on to others,
a characteristic of the ideology of oppression,
negates education and knowledge as processes of inquiry"

"Education must begin with the solution of the teacher-student
contradiction, by reconciling the poles of the contradiction
so that both are simultaneously teachers and student"
Freire (1996: 53)

Liberatory education encourages learners to challenge and change the world, not simply uncritically adjust themselves to it. The purpose of liberatory education is to establish a shared responsibility between learners and tutors/facilitators.

Any new courses have emerged that did not previously exist neither on the TNA or as a course offered by any organisation as far as CV is aware. Through the use of the TNA, at training needs meetings, discussion can also centre round the types of courses other CV learners from all over Renfrewshire are or have participated in. People start to talk about what they feel would help them in their group or volunteer role, this often results in new training or workshop ideas emerging. Through informal discussion, participants find out about various courses taking place, discovering that courses are designed in consultation with CV participants to suit their needs. Participants may not realise that courses are customised to suit participant's needs until a group or one to one discussion with the CAT Officer is entered into. Empowerment can result from liberatory learning. Building an individual or group's knowledge helps them to advance placing them in a better position to sustain their own development. Diverse or customised training and development recognises that people know what they want to do and why.

Identifying and Removing Barriers to Learning

The following section will examine CV's analysis tools and their use from first contact with participants at the TNA stage through to Mid course and End of course evaluations highlighting some of the discussions between the CAT Officer and individual participants and the group as a whole. It will look at child care issues, the flexibility of learning hours and literacy needs/support. It will further examine how unconventional teaching styles are adopted. Smaller learning groups out with the main group and how this helps to support CV participants through peer support will be discussed.

The TNA form asks participants to identify what day/time is most suitable for them to participate, if they require additional needs support or childcare with special needs. It is not always as easy as organising a crèche for participant's children. Some children need familiar surroundings and it may be necessary to negotiate a place at the nursery they are already attending. The CAT Development Officer, talks over the TNA form with the group, going through it a section at a time, this helps the Officer to become discretely aware of people who are uncomfortable with forms. The TNA has a section to inform the CAT Officer of how long it has been since the person completing the form has taken part in education or training. The CAT Officer is aware that some people prefer to have a one to one meeting to discuss any fears they may have i.e. negative learning experiences in the past or a need for literacy support.

Case Studies

The following case studies will look at diversity, barriers to learning and working in partnership with other agencies:

Case Study 1

The groups will be known as group 'A' and 'B', group 'A' work as volunteers on behalf of their local community, organising events such as gala days and small shot day. Group 'B' are volunteers with a group for up to 50 local children aged 5 – 12yrs old.

Volunteers from both groups encourage children to take part in celebrations in their community. Along with gala days and 'small shot' day they also organise Burns Suppers, Valentines Day, and Halloween celebrations to include the children. During a TNA meeting volunteers asked for workshops that would teach them how to make Mardi Gras type creations that they could involve the children in from the construction stage. They made a very large Loch Ness Monster among other creations. The point is that Nessie was created by local people using new skills. Nessie comes out to celebrate on many occasions from Burns Night to the local Gala Day. Nessie gets dressed up in tartan for Burns night and has been seen with a severed leg hanging from her mouth at Halloween. The children involved in what has now become a local custom are very proud of Nessie.

Case Study 2

Local volunteers from various community led and Renfrewshire council led youth clubs felt they would benefit from youth work training. The local college in consultation with groups and the CAT developed a new SQA accredited course an 'Introduction to Youth Work'. Although not part of the accreditation, an arts and crafts and hall game elements was added to the course at the participant's request. The course was put together and delivered on a Sunday locally again at participant's request. Childcare, a buffet lunch and transport were provided for participants.

The course tutor was aware that learning had to be pitched at the right level to suit all participants. Literacy skills were taken into account; two participants were open about their limited reading and writing skills. Both of these participants also knew the majority of their fellow participants through volunteering together. In addition a smaller group of four participants met up for an hour a week to read and discuss the content of handouts etc. to people who required literacy support. They also used the small group setting to plan their presentations.

The CAT Officer met up with the main group every three weeks to carry out reviews throughout the duration of the course. Participants within the smaller group that required literacy support had a weekly meeting with the CAT Officer to give them added support and to ensure that they fully understood course requirements.

During a mid course review one young man in his late teens when asked 'in relation to the youth work course '*is there anything that you can do now that you couldn't do before?*' He answered quite candidly '*Aye I can turn up on time and learn something and I don't feel stupid.*' Participants who had difficulty putting their words on paper due to limited literacy skills were asked questions on the course by the course tutor. Their answers were recorded on DVD and this was accepted as proof of learning rather than the traditional essay or report. This course has been run twice by CV training both times on a Sunday. There is such a demand for this course by local youth work volunteers that CV training will be running future youth work courses.

A mid course review is carried out with participants of all CV courses lasting six weeks or more; this is a review that helps to highlight any issues that participants may be experiencing with the course. All issues highlighted are input to the CV training data base and how the issue was dealt with is also input. This system of recording ensures that all issues highlighted at mid/end of course reviews are dealt with and not just recorded and forgotten about.

The CAT Officer acts upon issues highlighted by participants. An example of an issue with the youth work course was the time the course started. Before the course began all participants agreed on a three o'clock start this meant that they would finish at eight o'clock.

A few participants highlighted on their reviews that they would prefer to start earlier and finish earlier. This was put to the rest of the participants present on the day. Participants who were absent when reviews were carried out were contacted and asked if they were happy to change the time. Once this was agreed, the changes were recorded in the CV monitoring and evaluation system and the time was changed.

Case Study 3

The following case study will show how partnership working benefited local community groups NHS Dieticians and the CV training programme. Dieticians from the NHS approached the CAT to enquire if the CAT would contact community groups whose focus was health related. CAT Officers either visited or telephoned all health focused groups they knew of in the Renfrewshire area and invited them along to meet with the dieticians. Ten groups sent along a representative to the meeting. The dieticians explained that they were in the process of developing a 'Nutritionist's' toolkit and were hoping that community groups could assist them by taking part in a pilot programme.

The Nutritionist's toolkit training course was designed to be delivered by community facilitators as part of their group work sessions. After the initial six session pilot period participants were asked to give feedback on each of the sessions. Facilitators took action based on the feedback from participants and made alterations accordingly. Participants also gave course facilitators details of their experience of using the Nutritionist's toolkit with their groups.

Community group members also deliver Nutritionist's toolkit training to other groups in Renfrewshire. Examples of groups who have benefited from this training are an aerobics group, an elderly fitness group, a men only slimming group and a healthy eating group. Since the initial pilot period twenty community group representatives have taken part in the training.

Six of the original participants asked if they could be trained in healthy cooking to give community groups a chance to put the theory from the toolkit into practice. The CAT Officer set up a meeting with Have a Heart Paisley and the local college to see if they could develop a healthy cooking element based around the Nutritionist's toolkit.

The 'Cooking and Eating for Health' course was designed especially for use by the community in their groups. A Nutritionist's toolkit update session is arranged by CV training twice a year to keep community facilitators up to date with the latest legislation. Dieticians also want to ensure that the course is still being delivered in the community and ask for evidence of this.

Working with Partner Agencies

There are many examples of the CV training programme working with partner agencies. The CV training programme is informed by local Learning centres and community college via email of all courses offered in every community/learning centre in Renfrewshire. This is helpful if CV participants have asked for a specific course that they may have just missed out on due to the timing of their TNA meeting. To cut down on waiting time CV learners are offered a place in their local learning centre where they still learn in their own community. This option gives the CV training programme even more flexibility while at the same time building the capacity of locally based learning centres. CV learners taking part in non CV funded training are still given the same level of support. Training provided by other organisations i.e. suicide prevention training can be accessed by community groups where traditionally it was accessed through and delivered by statutory bodies. If required hall hires, hospitality, crèche and transport are organised by CV training. Mid/end course reviews, any issues raised and how they were resolved are recorded in the same way as courses fully CV funded.

Over the years CAT Officers have worked with groups who address many issues facing communities. Examples are Play groups, Parent's committees, Disability support groups, Tenant's and Resident's groups, Elderly groups, Fitness groups, Fishing groups, Healthy eating groups and many more, too many to mention. Because the CAT are in contact with these groups they can assist other agencies or organisations who want to make groups aware of services they can offer them.

Participant consultation before during and after the learning process (using TNA's Mid/ End of course reviews and follow up calls after 6months) is an ongoing monitoring and evaluation system that CAT use with CV participants. The CAT believes the cycle of action-reflection-action to be crucial to the success of the CV programme. Since the CV training programme commenced in April 2006 until December 2008, Two hundred and ten participants have completed accredited training to date with two hundred and thirty three participants completing non – accredited training. It should be noted that these figures do not take account of CV learners who have been signposted to other learning centres for some of their identified training with CV support. The above figures also do not account for learning led by community groups as a direct result of engaging with CV training.

It can prove difficult to coordinate the CV programme due to the amount of organising involved. Every person who has filled out a TNA is contacted, when their chosen course is being organised. Potential participants are contacted by phone, text message or email and asked for their preferred day, time and venue to enable them to attend training. If people cannot be accommodated; this can be for a variety of reasons. CV participants are asked if they wish to be held in the CV data base and contacted when the training opportunity arises again.

Course tutors are not always available especially during July-September when tutors of accredited courses are on annual holiday. During this period CV had a tendency to run non-accredited courses however alternative training providers are able to and have provided accredited training to the CV programme when necessary. After consultation with potential training course participants who have been contacted the CAT Officer has confirmation of how many people are available to train on their chosen course. The venue, crèche requirements, and course tutor are also confirmed verbally with participant and training providers at this stage. After a written quotation and confirmation is received from the course provider, crèche, hall hire and hospitality providers all this information is entered into the CV training data base and CAT finance spreadsheet. Evidence is gathered at each stage of the process, copies of quotations, invoices, signed register/s of participants, mid/end course reviews and letters to participants are kept in CV verification folders in training course order.

For most courses twenty letters are sent out a week to ten days prior to the course commencing, asking people who have not already done so to confirm their attendance and as written confirmation to people who have already been contacted by telephone . At this stage in the process the course is scheduled to go ahead because telephone contact has been made with over eight participants who have confirmed attendance. Some people who receive letters contact the CAT officer prior to the course commencing however many assume that their needs will be met automatically i.e. child care, special dietary requirements, transport or literacy support without consultation. This causes the CAT officer a lot of extra work contacting everyone who has received a letter and has not phoned to either confirm or decline a place on the course. Contact can sometimes prove problematic, especially when people are being relocated due to housing regeneration or changing mobile phone numbers for example. The CAT officer however knows how to contact people through community group networks again this can be time consuming. Every effort is made to contact potential participants to minimise the possibility that CV participants will miss a potential training opportunity.

Additional Outcomes

Forty people were selected randomly from the four hundred and thirty three participants who completed training with the CV programme. Participants were asked to answer a telephone survey questionnaire, survey questions were based on anecdotal evidence gathered by CAT Officers. Some CV participant's commented that if they had not participated in the CV programme they would not have had the confidence to undertake accredited training. Other participants were facilitating learning sessions in the community either as a volunteer in a group or an organisation. The CAT was also aware that five community group members had represented their group at an event or conference. The CAT team was informed by other agencies of CV participants who had found employment as a direct result of engaging with the CV training programme.

The graph below shows findings of the survey of forty CV participants who completed their training:

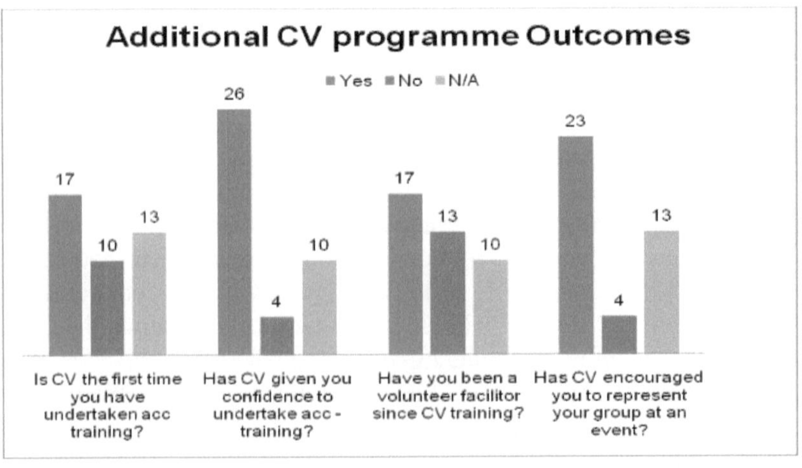

Conclusion

The CV training programme is successful for a combination of reasons. The CAT constantly updates their TNA and End/Mid course reviewing system to reflect the needs of the community therefore monitoring and evaluation is an ongoing process. Strong partnership networks with other agencies/organisations, community groups and individual volunteers is a crucial factor in the CV programme's achievements.

Reliable, dependable and professional tutors and facilitators who are willing to support learners with a variety of learning styles or literacy support needs and their willingness to work with the CAT and participants to modify the learning programme to meet their needs is also an important aspect of the success of the CV training programme. The most important reason for the success of the CV programme however is the community has ownership of their own training and development.

Commentary

This practice study illustrates very well the way that the current strong policy positions influences practice. Also evident is the underpinning statistical approach to defining both need and areas of need (data zoning). Overall, the work is well defined through its links to policy and reflects the importance of set targets and formal procedures.

It is interesting to see the discussion of Freire and liberatory education. Many workers would argue that the TNA process described here and the functional operationally focussed training delivered (food hygiene, book keeping, literacy support and basic IT) does not lead to the personal change and issue focussed work that is normally associated with liberatory education. What is interesting here is that the project in the study, and indeed many other workers, argue that it does.

What The Practice Studies Tell Us

> It is always the same: once you are liberated, you are forced to ask who you are.
>
> Jean Baudrillard

The 11 practice studies illustrate a range of contemporary community development related practice. Within each of the studies there are differing examples of practice, of modes of engagement with a variety of groups, and a diverse range of objectives, processes, outputs and outcomes.

Although there are often implied and sometimes stated ideological positions, it is remarkable that most of the work sits comfortably within a normative framework and provides little challenge to the status quo of power structures. A survey of community based work undertaken anytime from the late 1960's to the end of the 1980's would have shown far more ideological conflict with the state often appearing as the enemy, rather than the home / enabler / friend of community activity. Whether the increasing apparent domestication of community development is a good or bad thing depends upon your position. It could be argued that in becoming mainstream community development is now a more realistic enterprise and is in a position to get things done for local people. The counter argument is that community development has given up on struggling for meaningful social change and tackling structural inequality and oppression. The reader can take their own position here.

A close reading of the studies identifies a number of questions about the micro application of practice. These are critical questions and workers need to be clear about their answer to them to be effective in their practice. It is useful to discuss these questions in turn. In doing so we are discussing the general issues around these questions, not critiquing the descriptions of practice in the studies themselves.

Values

There would be few community development workers who would dispute that effective practice is based on a clear set of values. As we have noted the National Occupational Standards make a clear statement on values as the underpinning position for practice. They say that community development is concerned with addressing "*imbalances in power and bring about change founded on social justice, equality and inclusion*". In practice though it can often be that the value base is implicit rather than at the forefront of what workers do. How often do we discuss with groups what might be meant by these values and how to use them? Within groups we usually set ground rules but how often do we link them to values and associated wider social concerns? Do we consistently challenge gender oppressive acts, ethnic stereotyping, minor misuses of power and so on? Or, in order to help the group develop and avoid conflict can we sometimes ignore (collude?) with poor behaviours and attitudes. If we do this is it simply out of pragmatism or, are we just avoiding interpersonal difficulties and confrontation?

Difference

Most workers would say they value difference and diversity. The question is how far this perspective is active within our practice or is it just a passive position. We may confront discriminatory behaviour. But do we encourage groups to reflect on their own views, objectives and practice relating to ethnicity, gender, sexuality, religion and age. The spaces in which community development takes places are all structured with regard to these factors. Do we consciously try to make these spaces ethnically diverse, gender open and so on? Are we clear as practitioners when it is better to have a women only group or a black only group?

Underpinning theory

Without theory we are lost. Theory gives us explanations of why the world is like it is, why people do (and don't do) things, how to effectively organise, etc. It provides both a perspective and a framework within which to reflect upon our experiences and to learn from them. Often theories contradict each other. This is a good thing as no single body of ideas has a monopoly on truth. Critical engagement with theory forces us to work out what we believe, how we understand ourselves and the world, and provides us with a guide about what to do. Within this process we need to recognise that our positions must always be temporary and subject to re-evaluation in the light of new ideas and experience.

Theory is not helpful if it is simply a set of abstract ideas. Useful theory has to both relate directly to the world and be a product of it. Praxis, a term originally coined by Aristotle and modified by Kant and Marx is generally used today to denote the interlinking of theory and practice.

The question though is what theories are useful. Although there are many people who believe they have the answer, the reality is that everyone has to work at this and find their own theoretical position. It might be based upon a modernist view of the world or a postmodernist reinterpretation. It may for example be a late version of Marxism, communitarian or libertarian. It could instead focus on everyday life looking at, as we suggest above, the work of Lefebvre and de Certeau. It may be linked strongly as in some of the practice studies to Paulo Freire and maybe Gramsci. It can of course be a mixture of several of these things.

Some of the practice studies appear not to have any clear theoretical base underpinning the activities of workers. In this case workers simply act out mainstream social norms and policy objectives as if they are inherently good and implicitly neutral. But policy can never be neutral as everything is inherently ideological. They could be good, but if you don't subject the objectives and outcomes of policy to a theoretical evaluation, how can you know?

Reflexivity

Some workers see themselves as neutral in the process of change; that is they are in some respect external observers of what is going in a group or community. This is not the case. Whether we think it to be so or not, we are always subjectively involved in our social environment. We may try to create some 'objective distance' from what is going on to help us develop a perspective but we cannot totally remove ourselves from it. Even if we could we would not observe the events taking place with neutrality. We are, after all, human with our own viewpoints, ideals, prejudices and preferences.

Community workers need to consciously link theory and values in their reflection on practice. This is not just about considering a piece of work and evaluating what worked, what didn't and the lessons that can be learnt from the experience. It is also about going a step further and recognising yourself in the process and exploring the effect the experience has had on you, how it may affect what you decide to do next, and your impact on the process of change.

Bureaucracy and the local state

Many of the practice studies were situated within the work of a local authority, while others were based in agencies funded by them. Inevitably, the location, policy framework and often the objectives of a community development workers practice is linked to the operation of the local state or other bureaucratic organisation (e.g. Health Board).

The German sociologist Max Weber (see Camic 2005) suggested that the growth of bureaucracies under capitalism was inevitable, and would embed another form of domination upon society. As the Soviet Union demonstrated this was also to be true for societies based on state socialism. Ivan Illich (2005) has also explored how bureaucratic organisations have a tendency to operate in their own interest, rather than that of the people to whom they provide a service. At the top level this could be characterised as empire building, at the lower level just keeping within the rules and not annoying senior management.

The limitations of the local state/bureaucracy model for delivering public services are increasingly apparent. For example

Huczynski and Buchanan argue that *"...in the twenty-first century the bureaucratic organisation will be incapable of responding sufficiently quickly to change and will not be using the innovative resources of its members"* (2001: 495). The experience described in several of the case studies also suggests that the way bureaucracy operates can be a hindrance rather than an asset for communities.

It is likely that in post industrial western societies this centralising model will be rolled back in favour of more diverse market driven forms of delivery. It is often said that the policy models of the USA come to the UK ten years later. If so we should be looking out for the growth of non profit organisation increasingly taking up the public service delivery role. The new Conservative – Liberal Democrat coalition that has taken power as this is being written may make changes in this direction.

Many community workers believe in the potential effectiveness of the local state and the moral rightness for it to be done this way. Any movement to a market delivery model would be seen by many as a threat. It is also an opportunity. How else can services be delivered, what might local communities want here, are there opportunities for local communities to build their own accountable organisations, how might initiatives around social entrepreneurship be explored? These are some of the questions community workers could engage with.

Structure, operation and support of community organisations

How should community groups be organised; as collectives, as free flowing open structures, as formal committees? By default community development workers now appear to see community groups as little bureaucracies. There must be office bearers, minutes, written constitution, AGM's and so on. When helping local people set up community groups how often do we ask them how they might want to organise themselves, or even offer different organisational models.

Formal office bearers and a written constitution are sometimes the way to go for a group with a particular objective that involves public money. Sometimes though formality is a barrier and what is needed is a more flexible and open structure. Learning circles for instance are an underused but powerful form of organisation.

Many of the workers in the practice studies were engaged, either directly or indirectly, in capacity building activities with community groups. This activity poses the same questions; whose capacity is being built, for what purpose, what are the parameters of the training, what is not in the training, who decides?

There is a lot of rhetoric around capacity building suggesting it builds skills and confidence, and promotes empowerment. In some cases it is claimed to be a transformatory experience. In practice capacity building is often little more than information giving, training in basic committee skills, orientation to pre set roles within partnership structures, plus some first aid/health and welfare sessions. Mostly these activities are pre produced and taken off the self to be delivered to community members. The sessions may be interactive in method but that does not stop them being a banked educational experience.

A Freirean process would start with reflection on what people were trying to achieve, identify with them what they already knew and what they felt they needed to know, draw on local and external knowledge, and develop a tailored range of learning specific to the expressed needs of the people concerned.

It is now conventional practice to monitor activity and evaluate what is being achieved. This is as it should be, but the question is how it is done and the effect of doing it that way. Is monitoring and evaluation just a way of checking that money is not misspent? Is it a way of ensuring compliance by community groups to the wishes of the supervising agency? Is it a reflexive process for all concerned? Who decides the parameters of what is monitored and how it is done? Are the community the object of the process or genuine partners within it?

What should be the relationship of a community group be to the local authority/partnership? Is it an autonomous entity that is free to work with formal authorities or not? Is it a client of an agency that employs the community worker? Is it a subcommittee of a partnership? It can of course be any of these things depending upon what the community group is trying to do. What should not happen is that the community group, and the imagination of its members is inevitably tied into the interests and activities of more powerful bodies as a default position.

Power

The discussion about community group structure, who decides how they are organised and what they do, is of course a discussion of power. To promote change we need powerful autonomous community organisations. The cynic might say that locking community groups into rigid ways of working, dependent upon local authority funding and with a tied agenda, is a way of limiting their power. In terms of Arnstein's ladder of participation there are few community groups operating at the top level of participation. There are not many either at the partnership level if we define this in terms of equality of decision making. Most community groups are subservient to the formal holders of power.

Knowledge

As Foucault (1981) pointed out power is based on knowledge and uses knowledge to further its own interest. When we organise community groups, explore problems, define issues and discuss option; whose knowledge are we using? Do community workers help community groups to critically explore the dominant idea of how society is and should be and help people question their current and potential lives? Or do community workers take the everyday common sense normative knowledge, which both created and perpetuates the status quo as given and accepted.

Our critical understanding that there are different sets of knowledge is important for community development practice. All community development takes place in varying degrees within a social policy context. Who wrote this policy, based on what knowledge and ideological position, what has been excluded from the policy, how might the people/families/communities on the receiving end view these policies? One of the key roles of a community worker is to promote this debate.

This takes us back to the discussion on ideology, theories and values. Community groups can both create their own local knowledge and tap into alternative knowledge that suggest a different world. Community development is based on the idea of social change for the better and for this to happen people must have a real belief in the possibility of change. The community workers job is to facilitate the transformation of this belief into action. If discussion and action are limited by the constraints of normative ideas and process, how much change can be achieved?

Ideas of community

Community workers need to have clear understanding of what they mean by community. We discussed at the start of this book that to be meaningful 'community' has to be based on how people define themselves, rather than as an administrative construct. Furthermore, it is important to identify the micro communities within a geographical area as they are the starting point to build networks, social capital and organisations.

However, communities are not simply an amorphous collection of people; they are comprised of individuals and families. In order to work with communities and to engage people in the process of change, we have to work with their different needs and perceptions. A community group member may also be a parent, a partner, a local worker. In terms of the activities they are involved in they may be service users, customers, clients, unpaid workers or volunteers. How we define people shapes our view towards them and affects how we respond. It is not good enough to just talk about the community or see people as numbers to be trained or organised. We have to see and respond to the individual person and their specific needs within the group context.

Action points

From the above discussion there are a number of critical questions for practitioners. Many workers will of course be thinking about and responding to these things already on a routine basis. But in managing the pressures of life it can sometimes be easy to let our standards of practice slip. It can be useful for workers to create their own check list check list of good practice. As a suggestion to start this list I would offer the following:

- Make our value base explicit in our dealings with individuals, communities and organisations.
- Don't collude with actions that are oppressive just because it makes life easier, avoids conflicts, or might undermine the group.
- Be clear about our personal underpinning set of theories, and be prepared to discuss, reflect on and modify them
- Be creative on organisational models and group structure. Make it fun.
- Explore opportunities for non profit or social entrepreneurship organisational solutions to local service problems

Finally, in Freirean practice there is a basic saying of *'trust the process'*. It is alright not to know where the work is going, for people to struggle in reflecting on their experience and in defining what they need. Creative work and change can only come out of uncertainly. If we are content to simply replicate old models of organisation, re-deliver old training packages, and pre-determine outcomes then nothing will ever really change.

Just to give Paulo Freire the last words, he wrote in the seminal Pedagogy of the Oppressed that *"to achieve.. praxis, however, it is necessary to trust in the oppressed and in their ability to reason. Whoever lacks this trust will fail to initiate (or will abandon) dialogue, reflection, and communication, and will fall into using slogans, communiqués, monologues and instructions. Superficial conversions to the cause of liberation carry this danger. Political action on the side of the oppressed must be pedagogical action in the authentic sense of the word, and, therefore, action with the oppressed."* This is where we must start.

Appendix

National Occupational Standards for Community Development Work

What is community development practice?

Community development is a long–term value based process which aims to address imbalances in power and bring about change founded on social justice, equality and inclusion. The process enables people to organise and work together to:

- identify their own needs and aspirations
- take action to exert influence on the decisions which affect their lives
- improve the quality of their own lives, the communities in which they live, and societies of which they are a part.

What are the Standards?

The National Occupational Standards outline clearly the skills, values and processes required for effective and appropriate community development practice. We need
to use these Standards with confidence to argue for values and processes to be integral to the work. The Standards applied to practice will ensure that community development impacts on poverty, racism and social exclusion in a way that empowers, enables and encourages participation.

Key Values

The community development process is underpinned by a set of values on which all practice is based. Community development practitioners need to relate these values to their roles and actions. There are five key values that underpin all community development practice:

- Equality and Anti-discrimination
- Social justice
- Collective action
- Community empowerment
- Working and learning together.

The National Occupational Standards support

- Community development workers and community activists
- Individuals and organisations adopting a community development approach in their work
- Employers of community development practitioners
- Community development education and training providers
- Funders of programmes and projects
- Development and delivery of strategic plans
- Evaluation of community development practice

Key Areas and Standards for Community Development Practice

The National Occupational Standards for Community Development Practice consist of seven key areas that between them contain 25 standards.

Key Area 1: Understand and practise community development, underpins all the other six key areas. They identify the roles that community development practitioners adopt within the process and outline the knowledge, understanding and skills needed to carry out the roles.

1 Integrate and use the values and process of community development
2 Work with the tensions inherent in community development practice
3 Relate to different communities
4 Demonstrate competence and integrity as a community development practitioner
5 Maintain community development practice within own organisation

Key Area 2: Understand and engage with communities

6 Get to know a community
7 Facilitate community research and consultations
8 Analyse and disseminate findings from community research

Key Area 3: Take a community development approach to group work and collective action

9 Support inclusive and collective working through community development practice
10 Organise community events and activities
11 Respond to community conflict
12 Support communities to campaign for change

Key Area 4: Promote and support a community development approach to collaborative and cross-sectoral working

13 Promote and support effective relationships between communities and public bodies
14 Encourage and support public bodies to build effective relationships with communities
15 Use a community development approach to support collaborative and partnership work
16 Apply a community development approach to strategically co-ordinate networks and partnerships

Key Area 5: Support community learning from shared Experiences

17 Promote and develop opportunities of learning from community development practice
18 Facilitate community learning for social and political development

Key Area 6: Provide community development support to organisations

19 Advise on organisational structures using community development perspectives
20 Plan and gain resources and funding for sustainability through community development practice
21 Strengthen groups using community development approaches and practice

22 Set up new projects and partnerships using community development approaches and practice
23 Use a community development approach to monitoring and evaluation

Key Area 7: Manage and develop community development practice

24 Supervise community development practitioners
25 Manage internal organisational development and external relationships to support effective

Source;
http://www.fcdl.org.uk/NOS_Consultation/Documents/NOSsummarypilot.pdf

References

Alinsky, S.D. 1969. **Reveille for Radicals**, New York: Vantage Books.

Alinsky, S.D. 1971. **Rules for Radicals,** New York: Vantage Books.

American Medical Association. **Healthy Men and Women. . Paths to Health Training Course Manual for Walk Leaders**. AMA

Armitage, A., etal. 1999. **Teaching and training in post-compulsory education'**, Buckingham: Open University.

Arnstein, S. 1969. A Ladder of Citizen Participation, **Journal of the American Institute of Planners,** Vol. 35: 4 pp. 216-224.

Baldock, J., Manning, N.& Vickerstaff, S. (ed) 2003. **'Social Policy',** Oxford: University Press.

Barr, A. Hamilton, R. Purcell, R. 1996. **Learning for Change**, London: CDF.

Barret-Lennard, G.T. 1998. Listening, **Person-Centred Review**, 3:4 Sage.

Bhatnagar. A. Ines. A. 1994 **Health and Health Care: The needs of women of Bangladeshi and Pakistani Origin in Edinburgh**. Nari Kalyan Shango and Lothian Health Promotion Dept

Bhopal. R. Last. J. Donnelly. P. 2002. **Public Health: Past Present and Future,** Stationary Office

Blair. S. et al. 1989. Physical Fitness and all cause mortality: A prospective study of healthy men and women. **American Medical Association**

Bromley, C. Curtice, J. 2006. **Attitudes to Discrimination in Scotland 2006: Scottish Social Attitudes Survey,** Edinburgh: Scottish Executive

Brookfield, S.D. 1987. **Developing Critical thinking: Challenging Adults to Explore Alternative ways of thinking and acting**, Milton Keynes: Open University Press.

Burls, A. 2004 **Ecotherapy in Practice and Education**. Anglia Polytechnic University, Chelmsford www.openspace.eca.ac.uk/conference/proceedings/PDF/Burls.pdf

Camic, C, (ed). 2005. **Max Weber's Economy and Society: A Critical Companion**. Stanford University Press

Cohen, A. 2003. **The Symbolic Construction of Community**, London: Routledge

Craig. et al 2005. **The paradox of compact**, London Home Office

Craig. 2006. **The Engagement and support of Black and Minority Ethnic voluntary and community organisations in North Yorkshire**, Easingwold: NYFVO

Dailly, M. 1992. **Empowering users: a case studies on participation in service management by physically disabled people in Glasgow: Paper 11**. Glasgow: Gulbenkian Fellowship.

de Certeau, M. 1984. **The Practice of Everyday Life**, trans. Steven Rendall, Berkeley: University of California Press,

Drysdale, J. Purcell, R. 2001. **Reclaiming the Agenda: Participation In Practice A Handbook for Community Development Workers,** Bradford: CWTC

Evans, E. 1992. **Liberation Theology, Empowerment Theory and Social Work Practice with the Oppressed**, International Social Work, 35

Field, J. 2003. **Social Capital**, Routledge, London

Freire, Paulo. 1996. **Pedagogy of the Oppressed**, Harmondsworth,: Penguin

Foucault, M. 1981. **The History of Sexuality, vol 1**, Harmondsworth,: Penguin

Friedmann. J. 1992. **Empowerment: The politics of alternative development**, Oxford : Blackwell Publishers LTD.

Gauntlett, D. 2007. **Creative Explorations: New Approaches to Identities and Audiences**, Routledge

Glasgow Culture and Sport. 2008. **About Us**. retrieved May 25, 2009, from http://www.csglasgow.org/aboutus/

Gordon, Uri. 2008 **Anarchy Alive –Anti Authoritarian Politics from Practice to Theory,** Pluto Press

Gramsci, A. 1971 **Selections from the Prison Notebook**, ed by Hoare Q and Smith G, London: Lawrence and Wishart

Hannigan, T. 2005. **Managment Concepts and Practices**. 4th ed. Prentice Hall

Haughey, D. 2009 at: http://www.projectsmart.co.uk/smart-goals.html

Henderson, P. Thomas, D. 2002. **Skills in neighbourhood Work**, London; Routledge and Kegan Paul

HMIO (Education) 2006. **How good is our community learning and development**? retrieved April 14, 2009, http://www.hmie.gov.uk/documents/publication/hgiocld.pdf_

Hope, A. Timmel, S. 1995. **Training for Transformation**, London: ITDG Publishing

Hope, A. Timmel, S. 2003. *Training for Transformtion: A Handbook for Community Workers.* London: ITDG Publishing

Huczynski, A. Buchanan, D. 2001. **Organizational Behaviour**, Prentice Hall

IACD. 2009. **Measuring What Matters: Conference Report** http://www.iacdglobal.org/en/publications/iacd-publications/measuring-what-matters

Ife, J. 2002. **Community Development: Community-based alternatives in an age of globalisation**, Malaysia: Persons Education Australia PTY LYD

Illich, I. 1990. **Tools for Conviviality**, London: Marion Boyers

Illich, I. 1997 Needs, in Sachs W**, The Development Dictionary,** London: Zed Books

Illich, I. 2005. **Disabling Professions**, London: Marion Boyars

Jeffs, T. Smith, M. 1996. **Informal Education: conversation, democracy and learning**. Nottingham: Educational Heretics Press

Jones, M. 2006 **The American Pursuit of Unhappiness - Gross National Happiness (GNH) - A New Socioeconomic Policy** http://www.iim-edu.org/grossnationalhappiness/

Kolb, D. 1984. **Experiential Learning: Experience as the Source of Learning and Development**, Prentice Hall, summary at http://www.businessballs.com/kolblearningstyles.htm

Labonte, R., Featherson, J. & Hills, M. 1999. A Story Dialogue Method for Health promotion, knowledge, development and evaluation, *Journal Health Education. Research* Vol. 14:11 pp39-50.

Ledwith, M. 2005. **Community Development: a critical approach**, Policy Press

Lefebvre, H. 2008. **The Critique of Everyday Life** *vols 1-3*, Verso

LLUK. 2008. **National Occupational Standards for Youth Work**.

LLUK 2010. **National Occupational Standards for Community Development**

Lothian NHS. 2008. **Strategic Action Plan on Minority Ethnic Health: Being fair for all in the NHS**

Macionis, J. Plummer, K. 2005. **Sociology**, Persons Education LTD.

Maslow, A. 1943. A Theory of Human Motivation, **General Psychological Review**, 50

Mayo, P. 1999. **Gramsci,Freire and Adult Education-Possibilities for Transformative Action**, London: Zed Books Ltd.

Mays, R. Smith, V. & Strachan, V. 1999. **Social Work Law (Scotland)**, Edinburgh: W. Green & Sons LTD.

McKnight, J. Kretzmann, J. http://www.regdev.govt.nz/quotes/index.html#participation, cited 08/06/2009,

Mills, C Wright. 1959. **The Sociological Imagination**, Harmondsworth: Pelican

PAULO. 2003. **National Occupational Standards for Community Development Work**, at: http://www.fcdl.org.uk/publications/documents/nos/StandardsSummary%20feb08.pdf

Purcell, R. 2005. **Working in the Community: perspective for change**, North Carolina: Lulu Press

Rethinking Development Conference 2005 http://www.gpiatlantic.org/conference/

Scottish Executive 2004, **Working and Learning Together to build stronger communities**, Scottish Executive, Edinburgh.

Scottish Government. 2006. **How Good is our community learning and development 2: Self evaluation for quality improvement.** Livingston. HMIE

Scottish Government, 2007. LEAP: **A Manual for Learning Evaluation and Planning in Community Learning and Development:** Revised Edition, Crown Copyright, Edinburgh. Available on-line:
http://www.scotland.gov.uk/Publications/2007/12/05101807/1

Shor, I., & Freire, P. 1987. **Pedagogy of Liberation**, London: McMillan.

Skinner, S. 1997. **Building Community Strengths. A resource book on capacity building,** London: Community Development Foundation

Tett, L. 2006**. Community Education, Lifelong Learning and Social Inclusion**, Dunedin Academic Press

Tight, M. 1966. **Key concepts in Adult Education and Training**. London: Routledge.

Thompson, N. 1998. **Anti Discriminatory Practice**, Palgrave Macmillan

Tuckman, B. 1965. Developmental sequence in small groups, **Psychological Bulletin**, 63

Twelvetrees. A. 1976) **Community Associations and Centres: a comparative study**. Glasgow: Pergammon Press.

Twelvetrees, A. 2002. **Community Work**.. Hampshire: Palgrave

White, A. 2007. **A Global Projection of Subjective Well-being: A Challenge To Positive Psychology**? University of Leicester

Zangmo, T. **Psychological Wellbeing Survey Report,** The Centre for Bhutan Studies http://www.grossnationalhappiness.com/surveyReports/psychological/psycho_abs.aspx?d=pw&t=Psychological%20Wellbeing

www.ingramcontent.com/pod-product-compliance
Ingram Content Group UK Ltd.
Pitfield, Milton Keynes, MK11 3LW, UK
UKHW041945190726
13854UKWH00004B/1806

9 781446 139080